APPLIED DECISION MAKING FOR NURSES

APPLIED DECISION MAKING FOR NURSES

JO ANN GAROFALO FORD, R.N., M.S.

Associate Professor of Nursing,
California State University at Long Beach

LOUISE N. TRYGSTAD-DURLAND, R.N., M.S.N.

Formerly Assistant Professor of Nursing,
California State University at Long Beach

BOBBIE CREW NELMS, R.N., M.N.

Associate Professor of Nursing,
California State University at Long Beach

THE C. V. MOSBY COMPANY

ST. LOUIS • TORONTO • LONDON   1979

The C. V. Mosby Company
11830 Westline Industrial Drive, St. Louis, Missouri 63141

Library of Congress Cataloging in Publication Data

Ford, Jo Ann Garofalo, 1948-
   Applied decision making for nurses.

   Bibliography: p.
   Includes index.
   1. Nursing ethics.   2.   Nursing—Decision
making.   I.   Trygstad-Durland, Louise N.,
1940-   joint author.   II.   Nelms, Bobbie
Crew, joint author.   III.   Title.
RT85.F67   174′.2   78-15713
ISBN 0-8016-1624-7

C/CB/CB   9   8   7   6   5   4   3   2   1   02/C/219

PREFACE

Decision making is seldom taught formally. Primarily, nurses have learned decision making experientially on an individual basis. The new state nurse practice acts and the expanded roles of the nurse demand increased responsibility and accountability. Many of the nurse's responsibilities necessitate nursing judgment and decision making. For this reason, it is important that nurses be deliberately and systematically taught a decision making process.

This textbook integrates values clarification and decision making. The major focus is on clinical nursing decisions. However we conceptualize values to be an omnipresent aspect of decision making; awareness of these values facilitates rational decision making. Therefore, personal values are first examined and clarified, and then utilized as the foundation for learning a process of decision making. Each chapter begins with behavioral objectives, followed by a description and theory base for the chapter topic. Examples are given to clarify the topic. Numerous application exercises are included to reflect a variety of clinical areas and levels of nursing practice.

Written for nurses and all levels of nursing students, this book can be used by any individual nurse or group of nurses. It is appropriate for classroom use.

Jo Ann Garofalo Ford
Louise N. Trygstad-Durland
Bobbie Crew Nelms

CONTENTS

APPLIED DECISION MAKING FOR NURSES

1 INTRODUCTION TO DECISION MAKING

BEHAVIORAL OBJECTIVES

After completing the activities in this chapter you will be able to:

- Reflect on your own decision making to determine the components and process which you most often use.
- Discuss the rationale for learning a decision making process.
- Briefly describe the components of the decision making process as presented.

AWARENESS OF OWN DECISION MAKING PROCESS

The practice of nursing requires many decisions each day. The methodology for making these decisions varies greatly from nurse to nurse; some nurses have learned decision making through observation of others, some have learned decision making through successful and unsuccessful experiences of their own. When faced with the need to make a decision a variety of behaviors are possible: some nurses rely on intuition, some behave randomly, some rely on another person to make the decision, while others utilize a systematic process. All of these possible responses to the need for a decision may be made with or without awareness.

If you are considering learning a decision making process, it will be helpful to know how this process is similar to and how it is different from the process you already utilize. Knowing how the newly learned process would alter the present decision making process can aid in choosing whether or not to learn the new process.

Consideration of your current decision making process requires awareness of this process. This awareness can be gained through such activities as those at the end of this chapter, and also through reflection on your process at this moment.

1

The following questions are intended to help you reflect on your present decision making patterns.

1. Are you presently aware of how you make decisions?
2. Do you usually make decisions before beginning a task or at some point during the task?
3. Are you aware of making decisions before they are made, while they are being made, or after they are made?
4. Are you comfortable with the majority of your decisions?
5. Are you aware of commonalities between the decisions you make?
6. Do nursing decisions trouble you? If so, can you say why? What types of nursing decisions cause you difficulty?

RATIONALE FOR LEARNING A DECISION MAKING PROCESS

With expanded roles and functions in nursing, nurses are making more and more complex decisions than ever before; and nurses are responsible and accountable for these decisions.

A frequent concern in nursing is collecting and evaluating data in order to arrive at a sound decision. The decision making process presented here provides a means for organizing and analyzing information and choosing objectively from alternatives. These skills are essential to making a rational decision.

This process can be utilized individually or in groups. Nurses work alone and in groups and need to make decisions in both contexts.

Learning this decision making process will facilitate making decisions which are congruent with personal values and have a strong possibility of meeting individual objectives. This fulfills the desire to feel comfortable with and related to decisions.

This process is applicable not only to nursing decisions but also to all types of personal decisions. A sense of freedom in personal and professional life is promoted through experiencing choices and making decisions.

OVERVIEW OF THE DECISION MAKING PROCESS

The first portion of this process has as its focus the study of values, with emphasis on how they influence perception and action and determine decisions. Major sources of values and the ways in which values are learned are discussed. In this section you will have the opportunity to identify some of the values learned from a social context and possible changes occurring in those values. A description of behaviors indicative of clear and confused values is also included. The valuing process is described, and you are encouraged to analyze your values according to the valuing process and then place them in rank order. A discussion of institutional values and their relationship to personal values ensues. In concluding exercises in this section you are directed to focus on ways of dealing with, and resolving, value conflicts by integrating competing values.

Once values are clarified and ranked, one can proceed with the decision making process by developing behavioral objectives that reflect the ranked values. The basic elements of the behavioral objective are included in this section and an opportunity to practice writing them is provided.

An actual, or potential, threat to a stated objective results in the identification of a problem area. Problem identification depends on the individual's knowledge, skill, past experience, and situational characteristics. Thus, the next step in the process is to analyze the problem situation in order to make a concise problem statement.

The process continues with identifying possible options, which are possible solutions to the problem. Included in this section is a discussion of the role of creativity in option generation by using the techniques of lateral thinking, synectics, brainstorming, and quota setting. Those options that are not capable of fulfilling the behavioral objective are eliminated and the remaining options, now called alternatives, are analyzed according to three criteria: desirability, subjective probability, and personal risk. Desirability focuses on the decision maker's preference for an alternative. Probability looks at the likelihood that an alternative will be successful in meeting the behavioral objective. Personal risk taking has as its emphasis the amount of risk involved in the alternative. Each alternative is ranked according to all three criteria.

The next step in the decision making process results in the selection of one alternative, that is, the choice is made. To complete this process one must first reexamine the problem situation to rank the importance of desirability, probability, and personal risk in the situation. Once this examination is completed the alternative that best correlates with the problem situation ranking is selected. This alternative is the decision. However, the process does not end at this point; the final step is to evaluate the alternative chosen in terms of the decision making process. Evaluation focuses on the process, not the outcome of the decision. A good decision is one based on a systematic process.

Following the major content portion of each chapter is an example section that is designed to further clarify the subject matter through illustration. Some examples are chapter specific and others develop chapter by chapter as the decision making process unfolds.

Each chapter also has an activity section with application exercises that provide you with the opportunity to master the content in each section as well as practice the decision making process sequentially. The last chapter is devoted to the application of the total decision making process; several clinical situations are described, and you are directed to make decisions utilizing all components of the process.

The epilogue acknowledges that the book does not cover all possible facets of decision making. A brief discussion of patient involvement in the decision making process, teaching the decision making process, and decision making in groups is included.

The process may at first seem long and awkward, but with time and practice you will find the results beneficial. This book will enable the active learner to make systematic decisions based on clear personal values.

STEPS IN THE DECISION MAKING PROCESS

1. Value
   a. Identification
   b. Clarification
   c. Rank ordering
2. Behavioral objective formation
3. Problem identification and statement
4. Option
   a. Generation
   b. Screening
5. Alternative
   a. Analysis: desirability, probability, personal risk
6. Problem situation
   a. Analysis: desirability, probability, personal risk
7. Decision
8. Evaluation

ACTIVITIES

These activities are designed to help you become aware of your current decision making process.

ACTIVITY 1

How far are you going to read in this book today? Have you decided? If you have decided: Did you decide before you began reading? Did you decide after you began reading? Were you aware of making a conscious decision? When? List the considerations upon which the decision was based:

External factors	Internal factors
(e.g., class assignment)	(e.g., your interest)

Are external and internal factors equally important or is one more important than the other? Are you comfortable with your decision? If you have not decided: Are you aware of choosing not to decide? Do you expect to make a decision? If so, what external and internal factors will likely influence the decision? When will you decide? If not, upon what basis will you cease reading?

ACTIVITY 2

Consider your decision of what to wear today. Were you aware of making a conscious decision? Did you decide before you began getting dressed or as you began getting dressed? List the considerations upon which the decision was based:

External factors   *Internal factors*
(e.g., what was clean)   *(e.g., how you wished to appear)*

Are external and internal factors equally important or is one more important than the other? Is this usually true? Are there any external or internal factors which you wish you had considered? Are you comfortable with your decision? What commonalities exist between this decision and the decision of how far to read in this book today?

ACTIVITY 3

Consider a nursing decision which you made in the past couple of days. State the decision. Were you aware of making a conscious decision? When? Was the decision made before implementation or during implementation? List the external and internal factors which influenced the decision:

External factors   *Internal factors*

Did you overlook any important considerations? Are you comfortable with the decision? Would you make the same decision again? What are the commonalities between this decision and the decisions in activities 1 and 2?

ACTIVITY 4

Consider a nursing decision which was troublesome to you. State the decision. Were you aware of making a conscious decision? At what point were you aware of the decision? When did you make the decision—before or during implementation? List the external and internal factors which influenced the decision:

External factors   *Internal factors*

What other factors would you consider if you had to make the decision again? Are you comfortable with the decision? If not, list any discomforting aspects. What are the commonalities between this decision and the decisions in activities 1, 2, and 3?

ACTIVITY 5

State three nursing decisions with which you are comfortable and three which you consider troublesome. List commonalities and differences for the two categories. Consider when and how the decisions were made and the factors which influenced the decisions.

ACTIVITY 6

Review your comments in activities 1 through 5. List your assets and areas for growth in decision making.

Assets   *Areas for growth*

CHAPTER
2 ORIGIN OF VALUES

BEHAVIORAL OBJECTIVES

After completing the activities in this chapter you will be able to:

- Describe how values influence perception and action.
- Discuss the relationship of values to decision making.
- Discuss predominant sources from which values are learned.
- Discuss predominant ways in which values are learned.
- Given a situation, identify several underlying values in decisions made by others and identify underlying values in decisions made by self.
- Given a situation which describes the social context, describe prominent values of the social context which may be learned by modeling and direct experience.
- Describe your social context including culture and ethnic group of birth, decade of birth, values of parents, geographical location, economic status, religion, occupation, and peer values; identify some of the values inherent in your present social context.
- Compare some of your preferences and values with prominent values of your past social contexts.

If you purchased this book in order to learn objective decision making skills, you may reasonably wonder why it begins with three chapters devoted to the subjective topic of values. What is the relationship of values to decision making? Hawley and Hawley respond to the query in their statement, "Decision making is always based on value judgments regardless of how objective the criteria and whether the process is conscious or unconscious."[1] Rubinstein concurs that decisions are always value based.[2] Values are those beliefs and standards which we cherish as having intrinsic worth.

If you consider the decision to buy this book, you will note that it was based on values. If you purchased the book to learn decision making skills, you must value decision making skills sufficiently to invest time, energy, and money in learning

7

these skills. You may have bought the book not because decision making skills are valued but rather because the book is required for a course. In this situation, the purchase of the book reflects the instructor's values as well as your own. It is the course instructor who values decision making skills and you who value the course, either as an end in itself or as a means toward the end of completing an aspect of nursing education. If the book was borrowed rather than purchased, then values regarding learning are reflected, as well as values regarding economic restraint.

THE ROLE OF VALUES IN DECISION MAKING

Nursing decisions, both large and small, are based on values. The decision to become a nurse is probably based on many values, which may include interest, education, economic independence, mobility, and desired relationships with people. The decision to teach a wife about her husband's heart disease reflects values about teaching as an important aspect of health promotion. It also reflects values about the inclusion of family members in a patient's care. All nursing care is influenced by values.[3]

Even perception is influenced by values. Sitting down to talk with a patient whose posture and facial expression reflect sadness is based on values regarding responsiveness to sadness in others. But before the decision to sit down and talk can be made, the perception of sadness in another person must occur. This perception of sadness depends on the value placed on looking at people and learning to recognize subtle, nonverbal messages.

Values, then, may be described as the basis not only for a specific decision, but also the basis for those elements which contribute to decision making. Values underlie all actions and decisions. Values also underlie perception. What is considered important and relevant is determined by values and what is considered important and relevant influences what is observed and how it is observed. Values influence one's entire concept of reality.[2]

To be unaware of the values upon which decisions are based is to be unaware of an essential component of decision making; it is a way of making blind or uninformed decisions, decisions to which the decision maker feels unrelated. Think back to when you have asked yourself "Why am I doing this?" and have thought, "This is not what I want to be doing." Chances are you made a decision to do something which was inconsistent with your values, or else you were not aware of how the decision and activity were related to your values. Either way, you feel unrelated to your decision and activity.

Recognizing the central role of values in decision making is the first step in utilizing values deliberately and with awareness. Values which are identified can then be explored and clarified. They can also be set in priorities. As the connection between values and decisions is recognized and as values are explored, clarified, and set in priorities, more deliberate and effective decisions emerge. The decision maker will feel more related to decisions which are consciously made on a value base.[1,4] Obviously, we value the awareness of values in decision making; this value underlies our decision to present a discussion of values in the first chapters of this book and exercises to promote awareness of personal values throughout the entire book.

LEARNING VALUES

Values and attitudes are learned through what is seen and what is experienced. Learned behavior is likely to be performed if the situation seems appropriate and responses to the behavior have been positive in some way. This is based on social learning theory which says that learning occurs in two major ways: observation and experience.

Learning through observation

In learning through observation, behavior is observed along with the setting in which it occurs and the response which it brings forth. When one observes the behavior of another person, one learns that the behavior is a possible behavior. Whether or not the behavior is enacted depends on influencing factors, the strongest of which is the occurrence of a positive response to the behavior, including one's own positive response to the behavior as well as the positive response of others. Other influencing factors include the situation or setting, other alternatives from which to choose, other values which are held, and the importance of the people responding to the decision maker.

Imagine seeing a nurse on a busy surgical floor sit down for ten minutes with a crying patient to listen to him and comfort him. The head nurse comes in and angrily says to her. "What are you doing? There are medications to be passed." Imagine another nurse behaving in the same way on another busy surgical floor. When she is back in the nurses' station checking medication cards the head nurse says to her, "I'm glad you could spend a few minutes with Mr. G. . . . . He needs our support." In both situations one learns that sitting down and listening are possible responses to a crying patient, and that this can occur on a busy surgical unit. Sitting down and listening to a crying patient is more likely to be enacted by the observer on the second unit because the response to the nurse observed was positive. The observer may sit down and listen to a crying patient on the first unit if she has already learned that being supportive to patients feels right to her regardless of feedback from the staff, or if she has learned that this head nurse makes many such negative remarks but that these remarks do not threaten her job.

Learning through experience

The second major mode of learning is through direct experience. In this case a behavior may occur randomly, intuitively, or after reflecting on the possibilities—thus a behavior is learned. Performing the behavior a second time depends on influencing factors. As with performing a behavior learned through observation, the response is the strongest influencing factor. In learning through direct experience the individual is the receiver of a response rather than the observer of a response. She directly experiences the positive or negative responses of self and others rather than seeing them received by another person. Other factors which influence performing the behavior include the situation, other available alternatives, other values, and the valuation of the people responding.

Imagine being in a classroom, with the teacher reading a patient situation. It is a new situation to which none of the students has been exposed. The teacher asks if anyone has ideas on how to respond to the situation. One student shares her intuitive response. The teacher looks at her with a frown and says, "I can't believe you said that. Don't ever let me catch you doing that—no response could be worse!" In this situation the student may learn something about this particular patient situation. She has surely learned something about sharing her intuitive responses with this teacher. She is not likely to share intuitive responses with this teacher in the future.

Imagine that, in the same situation, the teacher smiles and says to the student, "That's a frequent response. Let's role play the situation using that response and observe the outcome." In this situation the student will probably learn something about the patient situation and that it is safe, appropriate, and even helpful to share intuitive responses in this class. If later in the class two classmates say: "I was thinking the same thing, I appreciate your saying it", the student is probably even more likely to share intuitive responses in this class in the future.

Learning from social context

Learning about values begins early in life. Learning takes place in a social context, that is, the social setting with all of the factors which influence the social setting. A child's first social context is his family. The family not only reflects the values of the parents, but also some of the values of the cultural/ethnic group and the religious group to which it belongs. Family values will be influenced by the education, occupation, and socioeconomic status of the parents and by friends of the parents. The social forces of the decade, political experiences, and geographical location also influence the family.

The child sees the examples set by parents, siblings, and others in his limited environment. As the child begins to interact with these people he observes their behavior. He also experiences their values and attitudes through their behavior toward him and responses to him.

Think for a moment about the family with whom you grew up. Can you identify some of the value you learned through observation about money, the environment, education, women's roles, and leisure time? What did direct experiences with your family teach you about values in these same areas?

Families, of course, do not reflect isolated values; families reflect some of the values of their culture. Other institutions (e.g., schools, churches) also reflect values of the culture; these cultural values had to begin somewhere. Matson identifies the four main sources for the values reflected in middle American culture. These four value systems are survival, Greek rationalism, hedonism, and Judeo-Christian tradition.[3] The survival value system originated when biological survival was always in question. This value system holds survival of self and species as the highest priority in living. Greek rationalism values reason most highly and believes that both man and the universe are governed by reason. Hedonism values pleasure for self most highly. The Judeo-Christian tradition values each person as an individual—this is the highest priority. Other Judeo-Christian tradition values include fairness and justice for all and individual behaviors which are helpful, loving, and trusting. Elements from all of these value systems may be identified in one's self, family, and social context.

Changing values

Values, once learned, do not remain constant. As you thought over your family's values you may have been aware that you do not continue to hold all of these values. With continuing growth come changes and new learning. Values development is a lifelong process. Since it is a social learning process set in a social context, values are subject to change with new observations of others, with new experiences, and with new social settings. Social context changes often; every new home, new job, new friend, or new interest varies the social context. With these changes, new behavior is observed and new experiences occur. In this way, new values are learned, presenting the opportunity to choose, prize, and behave in accordance with them.

SUMMARY

Values are the basis for all decisions. Perceptions and actions are always guided by personal values. Actions which are incompatible with values feel foreign. For this reason, recognition of personal values is the essential first step in learning this decision making process. Recognition of the role of values in decision making allows deliberate and aware utilization of values.

Values are learned through observation of others and through personal experience within a social context. Because new observations and experiences continue throughout life, values continue to change.

EXAMPLE: Bill Warren

Bill Warren is a registered nurse who works nights in the emergency room of the community hospital in his home town. During the day he is a student at a nearby university.

At 1:00 A.M. the ambulance brings in a middle-aged Japanese couple from an automobile accident. The paramedics state that he is fine but she has multiple lacerations from being thrown through the windshield. She is in shock; internal injuries seem a distinct possibility.

Bill asks the emergency room clerk to call the physician on duty and he begins his physical assessment of the woman. Forty-five minutes later, after she has gone to surgery, Bill looks into the waiting lounge to find her husband. He is sitting expressionlessly on the sofa. Bill goes over and sits down beside him. "This must be hard for you."

From this example, many values can be observed while other values can be assumed.

A complex set of values probably led Bill into nursing and then into working in the emergency room of his hometown hospital. Some of these might include a preference for a setting requiring acute care skills as well as psychosocial skills that was close to home and a university, and a position which would interest him and offer hours compatible with further education. His demonstrated values in this instance are skill diversity, job interest, further education, and compatibility of work and education.

Bill's behavior after the ambulance arrived reflects not only values but also priorities in values. His actions reflect valuing appropriate delegation of tasks, assessment and intervention into life-threatening situations, and emotional support, in that order. Had his values been different, his actions would have been different. All of these values were learned by observation and direct experience. Bill's behavior reflects aspects of survival values, Judeo-Christian tradition values, American values, and nursing values.

Bill's response to the husband reflects the broad value of giving emotional support. It also reflects valuing individual differences and cultural differences. Bill understands that men of the Japanese culture are likely to be stoic. His knowledge of cultural behaviors and his knowledge of reactions which often accompany accidents allow him to perceive a need for emotional support where the verbal and nonverbal behavior does not provide the usual clues.

The hospital where Bill works obviously values emergency service. Values regarding the needs of those waiting are reflected in the presence of a lounge. The community obviously values paramedic service.

ACTIVITIES

These activities are designed to help you fulfill the objectives for this chapter. In completing the activities, you will be recognizing the values which guide the decisions and behaviors of yourself and others. You will also identify some of the factors which have influenced the formation of these values.

ACTIVITY 1

Helen Black is a community health nurse. Last Wednesday she visited the home of 6-year-old Sissy Hansen, whose mother had not brought Sissy back to the clinic for follow-up treatment of an infectious disease. The purpose of the visit was educational and to encourage the follow-up treatment.

When Helen arrived at the home at 1:30 P.M., she found Sissy home alone with her 7-month-old brother. Sissy said her mother was in school and would not be home until 5 P.M. Helen returned early Friday afternoon and encountered the same situation.

Helen returned to Sissy's house again at 5 P.M. on Friday to talk to Ms. Hansen. Helen's concerns on this visit included the follow-up treatment for Sissy, Sissy's missing school, and Sissy and her brother being left unsupervised for entire afternoons. During their conversation, Ms. Hansen promised to take Sissy to the clinic for follow-up treatment on Monday morning. Helen asked why Sissy and her brother were being left alone. Ms. Hansen explained that she was in a training program from 12 noon to 4:30 P.M. each day. She had Sissy come home at lunchtime to take care of her brother. Ms. Hansen said she could not afford a babysitter.

Helen talked about the availability of local day care centers. She explained the available child care financial assistance, which was part of the same program that was paying for Ms. Hansen's training program. Helen emphasized the need in young children for supervision and the illegality of leaving them alone. Ms. Hansen said she would immediately discontinue the practice; she promised to apply for additional financial aid and enroll her children in the child care center on Monday.

By Wednesday noon, Sissy had not been to the clinic and the child care center had not seen Sissy and her brother. Helen visited Sissy's home and found Sissy there with her brother. Helen called the protective services division of the county social services department. A social worker from protective services came to Sissy's home and took Sissy and her brother to a foster home. They would remain there until Ms. Hansen worked out specific plans with the protective services worker.

Identify the values which underlie Helen's decision.

Describe the action you would have taken in this situation.

Identify the values which underlie your action.

ACTIVITY 2

Janice works in a private, 40-bed, acute psychiatric unit with a milieu therapy program. As patients are admitted they are assigned to one of four teams. Each team has at least one registered nurse and one nursing assistant on the day and evening shifts. Staff are consistently assigned to the same team.

Staff on the unit includes registered nurses with masters degrees, baccalaureate degrees, and associate of arts degree preparation. Also present are psychiatric social workers, occupational therapists, recreational therapists, psychiatric technicians, and nursing assistants. Most of the professional staff members have a particular preference for the theory base they utilize in individual and group therapy. At least five different theoretical bases can be identified as being utlized by staff. Staff includes both men and women, representing many ethnic backgrounds. Most of the staff have worked together for over two years. Staff members are very supportive to one another and frequently share personal and professional concerns.

Patients are admitted voluntarily with a variety of problems, including neurosis, psychosis, character disorders, and substance abuse. The age range is 15 to 80 years. Patients represent many cultural and ethnic backgrounds and have varied economic status. Most pay through private insurance or Medicare.

There is no set length of stay, but the hospital has a utilization review after 21 days. Visitors come nightly between 6 P.M. and 8 P.M.

Describe values which can be observed in the social context.

Describe your own social context including cultural and ethnic group of birth, decade of birth, values of parents, geographical location, economic status, religion, occupation, and peer values.

Identify prominent values in your social context.

ACTIVITY 3

Directions: Use form I to complete A through D and form II to complete E through H.

A. On form I list twenty things you love to do.*

*Adapted from "Values clarification: a handbook of practical strategies for teachers and students" by Sidney B. Simon, Leland W. Howe and Howard Kirschenbaum, copyright © Hart Publishing Company, Inc. 1972, New York.

FORM I. TWENTY THINGS I LOVE TO DO*

	P	C	F
1.			
2.			
3.			
4.			
5.			
6.			
7.			
8.			
9.			
10.			
11.			
12.			
13.			
14.			
15.			
16.			
17.			
18.			
19.			
20.			

B. In the column marked "P" check those items which would likely appear on a list made by your parents.

C. In the "C" column check those items which you believe are very frequently enjoyed by people from your cultural background.

D. In the "F" column check those items which would likely appear on the lists of your closest friends.

E. Draw a line through any activities that have not been performed in the past year.

F. Complete form II.

*Adapted from "Values clarification: a handbook of practical strategies for teachers and students" by Sidney B. Simon, Leland W. Howe and Howard Kirschenbaum, copyright © Hart Publishing Company, Inc. 1972, New York.

FORM II. TEN VALUES IN NURSING FOR ME

	CO	P	C
1.			
2.			
3.			
4.			
5.			
6.			
7.			
8.			
9.			
10.			

G. In the "CO" column, check those items which you believe are shared by co-workers or classmates.

H. Check values your parents would share in the "P" column.

I. Check values representative of your culture in the "C" column.

J. Compare both forms and note similarities and differences between values. How do you account for differences?

K. Consider what influences your current values the most: parents, friends, co-workers or classmates, your culture, your past experiences, or your present experiences.

REFERENCES

1 Hawley, R. C., and Hawley, I. L.: Human values in the classroom: a handbook for teachers, New York, 1975. Hart Publishing Co., pp. 210, 211.

2. Rubinstein, M. F.: Patterns of problem solving, Englewood Cliffs, N.J., 1975, Prentice-Hall, Inc., pp. 474, 476.

3. Matson, H. N.: Values: how and from where? Nursing Digest, September, 1974, pp. 36-38, 46.

4. Smith, D. W.: The effect of values on clinical teaching. In Williamson, J. A., editor: Current perspectives in nursing education, St. Louis, 1976, The C. V. Mosby, Co., p. 93.

3 CLARIFYING PERSONAL VALUES

BEHAVIORAL OBJECTIVES   After completing the activities in this chapter, you will be able to:

- Compare and contrast the behaviors indicative of confused values and clear values.
- Describe the valuing process and its expected outcome.
- Identify selected personal values and rank them in importance.
- Analyze stated values and personal behavior to determine whether these values have been: freely chosen from alternatives after consideration of the consequences of each alternative; cherished and publicly affirmed; acted upon repeatedly and consistently.
- Make a clear statement of selected values.
- Practice the valuing process.

VALUES CONFUSION

Mary sits apathetically and expressionless in the back of the class, regardless of who is speaking or what activity is involved. She appears to have almost no energy to put into learning about nursing. During the clinical laboratory session, Mary's behavior is hesitant and uncertain.

Doris's behavior seems flighty. Sometimes she looks as apathetic as Mary but, more often, she looks interested and talks in class. She always wants to talk about her primary interest; however, that primary interest changes almost weekly. Her papers and projects remain unfinished as she pursues her new interests. In the clinical laboratory, Doris's nursing care is inconsistent. Her learning and application both reflect her rapid changes.

Jim is consistently active in class and his position is always the polar opposite

17

of that expressed by the teacher, Miss Mapes. Jim can be counted on to disagree with any decision made.

Miss Mapes is as consistent as Jim. Rules are important to her and are the guidelines for her life. The class bulletin says her class is held on Tuesday's from 8 A.M. to 10 A.M., and that is when it is held, come sunshine, hurricane or a world-renowned speaker giving a lecture on campus from 9:30 to 10:30! Miss Mapes is proud to uphold the standards she learned 30 years ago; everyone addresses her as "Miss Mapes" as she walks down the hallways in her crisply starched uniform.

Janice gets along well with Miss Mapes because she has figured out what behavior Miss Mapes considers appropriate for a student and that is how she behaves. Janice's behavior in chemistry is markedly different, reflecting Janice's alignment of her behavior with the stated expectations of the chemistry teacher.

Emmy is a staff nurse in the clinical laboratory setting. A drifter, Emmy goes from task to task and job to job without investment or any apparent direction in her life. Miss Mapes likes Emmy least of all the staff and cannot understand how Emmy can be in the same profession.

All of the individuals described here appear very different but they share at least one trait. The commonality is that all of them display behavior which Raths identified as indicative of values confusion. Raths states that being uncertain and unclear about personal values leads to a confused relationship with self and society.[1] This in turn leads to specifically identifiable behaviors including apathy, flightiness, uncertainty, inconsistency, drifting, overconforming, overdissenting, and role playing.[1]

Kirschenbaum notes that conflict or confusion in values usually occurs when a range of values is held by different people. These "value rich" areas include health, personal habits, work, leisure, male-female roles, race, poverty, family, and friends. Other areas heavily influenced by values include love, sex, religion, money, and politics.[2]

The potential for values confusion is high. As Matson states, our society continues to reevaluate and alter what is considered good or right.[3] Within the larger society, institutions, families, and individuals reevaluate and change values. Marked changes in laws reflect marked changes in values by the broader society. Women's status has changed from that of legal nonentities to that of people with a right to vote and a right to equal pay for equal work. Capital punishment, once viewed as the appropriate consequence for particular behavior, may now be viewed as cruel and inhumane punishment. Differences in values and laws from state to state, divided by invisible boundaries, are enormous. In one state possession of small amounts of marijuana is a felony, while in other states it is legally permitted. Abortion may be easily available or strongly condemned. Alcohol may be sold in the university cafeteria or be illegal in the entire county. Soft drinks in disposable bottles may be the best sellers in the store or may be illegal to sell. Under the state law regulating nursing, private practice may be acceptable or clearly illegal.

Each individual is bombarded by different values. Values learned by observation and direct experience will vary according to the models and the responders. Nursing students who have learned values from Miss Mapes will have difficulty adjusting to Carol, the open and flexible instructor of the following semester. Miss Mapes and Carol model different values and will respond differently to students demonstrating their own values.

VALUES CLARIFICATION

It is clearly not possible for everyone to have the same values. Even people within the same family will have some differences in values. Individuals with diverse backgrounds and experiences are more likely to hold widely differing values.

Although individual values differ, it is possible for individuals to be clear about their own values. One way of achieving this clarity is through the valuing process which combines choosing, prizing, and behaving.[1] The process of choosing has three components—freedom, selection, and consideration of the consequences. The choice must be a free choice. It is not free if one person has blindly adopted someone else's choice or has in some way been coerced in selection. The choice must have been made from more than one possibility, since choice means "selected from possibilities." Choice must include an awareness of the consequences of each possibility. If one has considered several possibilities but has not considered the outcomes of these possibilities, then one has not chosen. Choice involves choosing freely from several possibilities after considering expected outcomes for each.

Prizing the choice involves two components—private satisfaction and public satisfaction. Satisfaction with the value is not only experienced personally but also demonstrated publicly by the willingness to openly declare the value.

Acting also includes two components—translating values into behavior and behaving consistently. Holding values means demonstrating values through behavior. This behavior reflecting choice must occur not once, but repeatedly.

Raths' valuing process may be summarized as follows:

Choosing
1. Freely
2. From possibilities
3. After consideration of consequences of these possibilities

Prizing
4. Being happy with the choice
5. Being willing to affirm the choice to others

Acting
6. Behaving on the basis of the choice
7. Behaving repeatedly on the basis of the choice

The valuing process may be demonstrated in the selection of a nursing education. The value (becoming a nurse) would be chosen without pressure after consideration of other fields for which aptitude and interest exist and after evaluation of the consequences of these other choices. As a result of the choice, there would be personal satisfaction as well as public declaration of wanting to be a nurse whenever there is discussion focused on career selection. Repeatedly enrolling in nursing courses, attending classes, and fulfilling course requirements would reflect the consistent behavioral portion of the value.

A particular behavior does not always reflect one particular value. The behavior which demonstrates a specific value for one person may reflect another value for someone else. In the above example, enrollment of a student in a nursing curriculum reflects the value of becoming a nurse. For another student, similar enrollment may reflect a father's offer to pay for a college education only if nursing is chosen. The father's value is nursing, while the student's value is having her father pay for the education.

A student may think, "All of those behaviors are not essential to my holding a value. I value political involvement by nurses. I just don't have time to behave that way while I am in school." What has just been described is a value indicator.[1] A value indicator is to a value what a highway is to a destination—it is going in the direction of a value but is not yet a value. It has some of the components of a value but is not yet fully actualized. In this example, political involvement may have been freely chosen from alternatives after consideration of the consequences; the worth of political action may be publicly affirmed and this may bring satisfaction. However, the action component is not yet present.

Value indicators are excellent content for the application of the values clarifying process. The value indicators used may include goals, aspirations, attitudes, interests, feelings, beliefs, activities, concerns, and problems. With the values clarifying process, you can analyze progress in actualizing values.

After years of working with values clarification, Kirschenbaum developed his own definition of the valuing process, which includes five components: thinking, feeling, choosing and decision making, communicating, and acting.[2] The thinking component of the valuing process includes all of the learning and activities that promote more effective reasoning; for example, thinking on various levels, critical thinking, moral reasoning, and divergent and creative thinking. The feeling component includes learning to deal with feelings and developing a stronger self-concept. Choosing and decision making include skills in setting goals, gathering information, considering possibilities and their consequences, and identifying influencing factors. Kirschenbaum describes the communication component as a continuing social interaction process, including the ability to send clear messages, listen actively, and resolve conflict. The acting component includes behaving consistently and skillfully on the basis of values.[2]

Raths' and Kirschenbaum's descriptions of the valuing process are somewhat different but compatible. Kirschenbaum specifically identifies particular skills in thinking, feeling, and communicating as part of the process. These areas are more implicit in Raths' work.

You may note that we have described values clarification as a basis for decision making. Raths includes the decision making process as part of choosing a value. Kirschenbaum describes learning decision making skills as an aspect of learning the valuing process. Obviously, these three viewpoints have many elements in common. The difference is one of focus. There is agreement on the importance of exploring values and learning decision making skills and on the interrelatedness of these areas.

Individuals achieve awareness and development of personal values by participating in the valuing process.[1] The outcome of the valuing process is different for each person because of the differences in values. Values clarification is not an attempt to teach particular values but is a process through which values are developed. As a result of choosing, prizing, and acting, you can develop a clear value and can make a clear statement of that value by using a subject reference and an action verb.

"So what if I learn the valuing process?" you may ask. "How will it help me?" Raths made clear statements about the gains from clarifying values. He said people with clear values can relate to themselves and their society in a satisfying, intelligent way. This will be evidenced by their being positive, purposeful, enthusiastic, and proud.[1] He further stated that students practicing the valuing process can expect to have more values, be more aware of their values, and have more consistent values.[1]

Kirschenbaum stated a consistent position. He described two objectives of values clarifying experiences: (1) becoming clearer about values held, and (2) developing one's own new values and value systems, which lead to purposefulness and commitment.[2] He defined the values clarification process as "an approach that utilizes questions and activities designed to teach the valuing process and to help people skillfully apply the valuing process to value rich areas of their lives."[2]

The general findings of research available at the time Raths published his book in 1966 supported his belief that students would become more purposeful and active as a result of values clarification.[1] Eight years later Kirschenbaum reviewed the values clarification literature and noted a growing body of research which supports Raths' predictions.[2] Research also supports the belief that values clarification leads to greater self-esteem[2,4,5] and growth in the direction of self-actualization.[2,6] Values clarification appears to foster belief in personal control over personal life.[7] Attitude changes include a more positive attitude toward learning,[4,5,8] while behavioral changes include more self-direction and initiative in classroom activities.[4,5,7] An increase in appropriate participation and a decrease in inappropriate verbal behavior was found.[9] The use of values clarification was also found to improve cognitive achievement,[10] decision making,[7] and reading comprehension.[1]

For many nurses, self-awareness is a value indicator that may become a value through values clarification. The process can be initiated by choosing the alternative of learning the valuing process with the expectation of becoming more aware.

Private and public satisfaction with enhancing awareness followed by repeated application of the valuing process and participation in values clarification activities will successfully actualize the value. In this way, it is possible for values clarification to assist nurses in developing purposefulness and commitment both personally and professionally. Naturally, the specific purpose and commitment will vary for individuals, reflecting differing values.

SUMMARY

Confusion about personal values is reflected by a confused relationship with self and society; such a confused relationship is characterized by specific behaviors, including lack of interest, inconsistent behavior, and attempts at consistency through rigid conformity or dissent. The valuing process is a means for achieving clarity about personal values. Within this process, one chooses values freely from possibilities after considering the expected outcome for each available choice. This choice of values is then prized, publicly affirmed, and acted upon repeatedly. Anyone who practices this valuing process can expect to be more aware of personal values and to hold more consistent values. This will be reflected in a more positive and enthusiastic attitude and more purposeful behavior. Research findings support these conclusions.

EXAMPLE: Jeanine

This example demonstrates a clearly stated value derived from the valuing process.

Jeanine values eating natural foods (clearly stated value contains subject and object references and action verb.)

Jeanine consistently selects and eats natural foods. (A value which is clear to the holder is acted upon repeatedly. It is also chosen freely from other possibilities after consideration of the consequences of these possibilities. The value is openly prized.)

When Jeanine began studying nutrition she became aware of the many different points of view on the subject. Different authorities stressed different aspects of nutrition. Jeanine considered the following possibilities and their expected outcomes.

Possibility 1: To eat as she had always eaten.
  Expected outcome: No expenditure in time and energy in learning new dietary patterns. Possibility that current good health would not be maintained if dietary patterns were indeed related to health.
Possibility 2: To eat fortified and enriched foods.
  Expected outcome: Time and energy expended in learning to recognize and buy these foods. Possibility of maintenance or nonmaintenance of health depending on the value of chemical enrichment and fortification.
Possibility 3: To eat foods which would maintain current weight.
  Expected outcome: No additional time and energy needed to learn this since she had already studied calorie contents. Maintenance of health to extent health and proper weight are related. Possibility that current health would not be maintained to extent that factors other than calories are related to health.

Possibility 4: To eat natural foods.

Expected outcome: Investment of time and energy in learning about these foods and finding markets which sell them. Expectation that health would be maintained and improved is based on new knowledge.

Jeanine has chosen the fourth possibility and believes the outcome will include improved health. She feels good about her choice and shares her convictions whenever the discussion topic is dietary patterns or health.

ACTIVITIES

These activities are designed to help you summarize the content of this chapter. (Keys for activities 1 and 2 are at the end of activity 2.)

ACTIVITY 1

Compare and contrast the behaviors of confused and clear values.

Confused values	*Clear values*
1.	1.
2.	2.
3.	3.
4.	4.
5.	5.

ACTIVITY 2

Describe in writing the valuing process and its expected outcome.

Key for activity 1

Confused values	*Clear values*
Apathy	Positiveness
Flightiness	Purposefulness
Uncertainty	Enthusiasm
Inconsistency	Pride
Drifting	Awareness of values
Overconforming	
Overdissenting	
Role-playing	

Key for Activity 2

The valuing process:
Choosing freely from possibilities and after consideration of consequences.
Prizing your choise; publicly affirming your choice.
Acting on the basis of your choice repeatedly.

Expected outcome: awareness of expanded, consistent values; increased satisfaction relating to self and society demonstrated by purposeful behavior.

The following activities focus on values clarification. They can help you to gain awareness of the beliefs and behaviors you prize and would be willing to proclaim in front of others. The activities are designed to help you consider different modes of thinking and acting, to weigh the advantages, disadvantages, and consequences of different possibilities. Also, the activities can help you analyze whether or not your beliefs and behavior are congruent.

ACTIVITY 3: ranking in importance*

Purpose: This activity helps you to recognize that identifying choices depends on values and consideration of consequences. It provides practice in choosing from identified options. If these choices are discussed in a small group, you will gain practice in publicly affirming your choice.

Directions: Rank your choices for the following questions. Use 1 as most preferable and 3 (4 or 5) as least preferable.

a. Whom would you prefer to marry? A person with:
____Intelligence
____Personality
____Sex appeal

b. Which would you most like to improve:
____Your looks
____The way you use your time
____Your social life

c. You've spent a great deal of time picking a gift for a friend. You give it to him personally. If your friend does not like the gift, what would you rather he do?
____Keep the gift and thank you politely.
____Tell you he does not like it.
____ Return the gift to the store without telling you.

d. What is the worst thing you could find out about your teenager? (Does sex make any difference?)

---

*Adapted from "Values clarification: a handbook of practical strategies for teachers and students" by Sidney B. Simon, Leland W. Howe and Howard Kirschenbaum, copyright © Hart Publishing Company, Inc. 1972, New York.

____That he has been shoplifting.

____That he has experimented with several kinds of drugs.

____That he has been or is promiscuous.

e. Which would you least like to be?

____Very sickly

____Very poor

____Disfigured

f. When you worry about a grade on an exam, what do you think about?

____Yourself

____Peers

____Family

____The teacher

____Graduate school

g. Which of these would be most difficult for you to accept?

____Death of a parent

____Death of your spouse

____Your own death

h. Which are you more concerned about as you grow older?

____Cancer

____Immobility

____Loneliness

i. Where would you rather be on Saturday?

____At the beach

____In the woods

____In a department store

j. Which would you be most likely to take a course in?

____Sex education

____Race relations

____Ecology

ACTIVITY 4: present life values*

Purpose: The ability to set priorities or place values and activities in order of importance depends on making choices from competing possibilities. This activity provides this practice.

Directions: Read the list of present life values and number them in order with number 1 being most important to you and number 27 least important to you.

*Adapted from "Values clarification: a handbook of practical strategies for teachers and students" by Sidney B. Simon, Leland W. Howe and Howard Kirschenbaum, copyright © Hart Publishing Company, Inc. 1972, New York.

PRESENT LIFE VALUES

_____ Make a new discovery

_____ Complete my education

_____ Achieve the goals of my religion (salvation, nirvana)

_____ Be at peace with myself

_____ Learn to resolve conflicts I have with others

_____ Have a close love relationship with another adult

_____ Have and rear children

_____ Be accepted by my parents for the person I am

_____ Accept my parents for the people they are

_____ Be in excellent health

_____ Change my appearance to be the beautiful person I want to be

_____ Live in a world at peace

_____ Understand human behavior

_____ Know myself

_____ Be aware of my own feelings

_____ Express my own feelings

_____ Live in a clean environment

_____ Develop close friendships

_____ Live a peaceful life

_____ Live an exciting, stimulating life

_____ Work/study part time so I have time for other important activities

_____ Have a challenging job even if it takes more than 40 hours a week

_____ Gain recognition, be an expert and authority in my chosen field

_____ Develop an active fantasy life

_____ Feel I have contributed to the well-being of mankind

_____ Travel at will, be free of commitments and responsibilities

ACTIVITY 5: values grid*

Purpose: This is an opportunity to check your alignment of desires with behavior. In activity 4 you indicated the five most important values for you. Remembering that the valuing process includes choosing, cherishing, and behaving, check these behaviors for yourself to see if you have listed value indicators or values. Directions: List your values, numbered 1 through 5, from activity 4. Put a check mark in each column that is true for you regarding the value named in the left-hand column.

*Adapted from "Values clarification: a handbook of practical strategies for teacher and students" by Sidney B. Simon, Leland W. Howe and Howard Kirschenbaum, copyright © Hart Publishing Company, Inc. 1972, New York.

Values	Chosen freely	From alter- natives	After consid- ering conse- quences	Happy with choice	Proclaim choice	Act on choice	Act repeat- edly
1.							
2.							
3.							
4.							
5.							

ACTIVITY 6: rest in peace*

Purpose: This is another opportunity for observing congruence between value indicators and behavior.

Directions: Fill in the form to complete your own desired obituary. Afterward, reflect on whether or not your current behavior is compatible with the outcome of life described in your obituary. For instance, leaving behind a circle of close friends and family suggests a life pattern of time and energy devoted to developing and maintaining relationships.

_____, age _____ died today of _____. He (she) is survived by _____ _____. Until death, his (her) principle endeavor was _____ _____. He (she) will be remembered by _____ _____ because _____ _____.

Notable contributions were made in the area of _____ _____. He (she) always hoped that _____ _____. He (she) was a member of

_____.

Flowers may be sent to _____ _____. In lieu of flowers please _____ _____.

ACTIVITY 7: values situation[1]

Purpose: This activity provides practice in choosing and prizing.

Directions: After reading the situation, answer the questions below. If possible, discuss the situation with a small group.

You are a mental health nurse working for the state in a crisis-oriented outpatient clinic. You have been excused from the clinic today to attend a one-day

*Adapted from "Values clarification: a handbook of practical strategies for teacher and students" by Sidney B. Simon, Leland W. Howe and Howard Kirschenbaum, copyright © Hart Publishing Company, Inc. 1972, New York.

workshop, "New Dimensions in Crisis Intervention," at the university. You will be one of several hundred in attendance. Crisis has been one of your interests for the past year. You have read extensively about crisis and attended two other workshops this year.

Under which of these conditions would you consider playing hooky today?

____ If you knew the important information from the seminar would be gathered and shared by the two other people from your clinic who will attend next week
____ If you knew you would not be caught
____ Under no circumstances
____ In the event of a family emergency
____ If a dear friend who lived 1500 miles away was in town only for today
____ If you believed you had earned a "mental health day"
____ If you drove past an outrageously good sale on the way to the seminar
____ Other (describe)

Discussion questions:

1. What values are reflected by your choice? Are they chosen freely from other possibilities after consideration of the consequences?
2. Would you share these values with anyone? With whom?

REFERENCES

1. Raths, L. E., Harmin, M., and Simon, S. B.: Values and teaching, Columbus, Ohio, 1979, Charles E. Merrill, pp. 4-6, 10, 30-32, 38, 110-111, 218.
2. Kirschenbaum, H.: Clarifying values clarification: some theoretical issues and a review of research, Group and Organizational Studies **1:**99, 100, 102-114, 1976.
3. Matson, H. N.: Values: how and from where? Nursing Digest, September, 1974, p. 46.
4. Covault, T.: The application of values clarification teaching with fifth grade students to investigate their influence on student's self-concept and related classroom coping and interacting behaviors, Unpublished doctoral dissertation, Ohio State University, 1973.
5. Guziak, S. J.: The use of values clarification strategies with fifth grade students to investigate influence on self-concept and values, Unpublished Doctoral Dissertation, Ohio State University, 1974.
6. Osman, J.: The use of selected value clarifying strategies in health education, J. School Health **43:**621-623, 1974.
7. Blokker, W., Glaser, B., and Kirschenbaum, H.: Values clarification in health education, Health Education, 1976.
8. Rutkowski, D. M.: The use of values-clarification strategies in chemistry classes to develop positive attitudes toward science, Unpublished master's thesis, State University College of New York at Oswego, 1975.
9. Wenker-Konner, R., Hammon, E., and Egner, A.: A functional analysis of values clarification strategies on the participation rate of ten fifth graders, Burlington, 1973, University of Vermont.
10. Barman, C. R.: The influence of values clarification techniques on achievement, attitudes and affective behavior in high school biology, Unpublished doctoral dissertation, University of Northern Colorado, 1974.
11. Precejus, E.: The effect of values clarification on reading comprehension, Unpublished doctoral dissertation, University of Pittsburgh, 1975.
12. From "Values clarification: a handbook of practical strategies for teachers and students" by Sidney B. Simon, Leland W. Howe and Howard Kirschenbaum, copyright © Hart Publishing Company, Inc. 1972.

4 VALUE CONFLICT

BEHAVIORAL OBJECTIVES

After completing the activities in this chapter you will be able to:

- Identify values stated by the nursing profession, bureaucratic systems, and your specific institutional environment (educational or service agency).
- Identify conflicts between professional and institutional values.
- Identify and discuss conflicts among professional and institutional values and your personal values.
- Describe possible responses to value conflict.
- Discuss your own most common value conflict responses.
- Discuss ways to resolve value conflict.
- Given a situation which describes the possibility of professional, institutional, and personal value conflict you will be able to:

    Identify the values belonging with each subgroup.

    Place the values in each subgroup in rank order.

    Analyze the extent to which you have freely chosen each value from alternatives after consideration of the consequences, and the extent to which these values are cherished, publicly affirmed, acted upon repeatedly and consistently.

    Integrate the values from all three subgroups into one list in rank order.

If you have chosen to be a nurse and to work or study in a institutional setting, you will experience value conflict. These value conflicts are predictable because three different sets of values will not be perfectly congruent: (1) each individual has unique personal values; (2) the professional associations of the nursing profession hold clearly stated values for nursing and educational institutions teach ideals for nursing, and; (3) each setting which employs nurses will have expectations of behavior which reflect the values of the employer. It is unrealistic to expect that these different sets of values will be in perfect harmony; it is realistic to expect to learn to identify and understand value conflict and then behave in accordance with personal values.

PROFESSIONAL VALUES

The two largest professional nursing organizations have stated standards for nursing practice. The National League for Nursing (N.L.N.) has developed a list of twenty-one nursing problems presented by patients:

1. To maintain good hygiene and physical comfort.
2. To promote optimal activity; exercise, rest, and sleep.
3. To promote safety through prevention of accident, injury, or other trauma and through the prevention of the spread of infection.
4. To maintain good body mechanics and prevent and correct deformities.
5. To facilitate the maintenance of a supply of oxygen to all body cells.
6. To facilitate the maintenance of nutrition of all body cells.
7. To facilitate the maintenance of elimination.
8. To facilitate the maintenance of fluid and electrolyte balance.
9. To recognize the physiological responses of the body to disease conditions—pathological, physiological, and compensatory.
10. To facilitate the maintenance of regulatory mechanisms and functions.
11. To facilitate the maintenance of sensory function.
12. To identify and accept positive and negative expressions, feelings, and reactions.
13. To identify and accept the interrelatedness of emotions and organic illness.
14. To facilitate the maintenance of effective verbal and nonverbal communication.
15. To promote the development of productive interpersonal relationships.
16. To facilitate progress toward achievement of personal spiritual goals.
17. To create and/or maintain a therapeutic environment.
18. To facilitate awareness of self as an individual with varying physical, emotional, and developmental needs.
19. To accept the optimum possible goals in the light of limitations, physical and emotional.
20. To use community resources as an aid in resolving problems arising from illness.
21. To understand the role of social problems as influencing factors in the cause of illness.*

The identification of these particular problems and the description of appropriate nursing responses to them reflects some of the values of the N.L.N. The implication is that individuals choosing nursing as a profession should prize these functions and repeatedly fulfill them. The identified problems indicate that the N.L.N. values cognitive skills of identifying, recognizing, understanding, and

---

*Reprinted with permission of Macmillan Publishing Co., Inc., from *Patient-Centered Approaches to Nursing* by Irene L. Beland, Ruth V. Matheney, Faye G. Abdellah and Almeda Martin. Copyright, Macmillan Publishing Co., Inc., 1960.

creating; affective skills of accepting; and psychomotor skills of preventing, maintaining, promoting, facilitating, and utilizing. These skills are used in responding to patient needs, including physical, psychological, interpersonal, social, environmental, and spiritual needs and the interrelationship of all these needs.[1]

In other words, if a nurse does not choose, prize, and utilize these skills in response to these patient needs, then she has a value conflict with the N.L.N. For example, if a nurse does not value spirituality for herself, she may not choose to respond to the expressions of spiritual questioning by 27-year old Steve Elmer, a newly diagnosed diabetic. She might refocus the interaction to the expression of his feelings as a result of his newly diagnosed diabetes mellitus. If she does not value the expression of negative feelings, then she might refocus the interaction away from the expression of anger about the diagnosis of diabetes to a discussion of the hygiene required in diabetes.

A nurse may or may not be aware of and uncomfortable with her value conflict with the N.L.N. Awareness and discomfort are relative to the situation. For example, the nurse who has interacted with Steve Elmer may attend an N.L.N. convention session which describes the ventilation of negative emotions toward the diagnosis of diabetes as essential before health teachings in relationship to diabetes can be accepted. At this point she might be uncomfortable remembering her behavior with Steve Elmer.

Alternatively, the nurse may be in a team conference with other secularly oriented nurses in a secular setting discussing ways to create more time for essential health teachings to the many newly diagnosed diabetic patients. She may remember refocusing away from nonessential topics involving spirituality and anger with Steve Elmer and feel pleased. She might share her refocusing as a way of protecting essential health teaching time.

The American Nurses Association (A.N.A.), in its attempt to define nursing, has established standards of practice based on nursing process. The focus on standards of practice indicates a value of competence in action. A.N.A. publications give the criteria for actualizing this value so that any nurse may align herself with A.N.A. values. That is, she may choose competence as her value, prize it, and repeatedly behave competently. She knows she is behaving competently if her actions are those described as factors for the standards.

For example, the nurse may value Standard III: "The plan of nursing care includes goals derived from the nursing diagnosis.[2]" This value will be reflected in her behaving according to the following assessment factors:

Goals are mutually set with the client/patient and pertinent others:

They are congruent with other planned therapies.

They are stated in realistic and measurable terms.

They are assigned a time period for achievement.

Goals are established to maximize functional capabilities and are congruent with:

Growth and development
Biophysical status
Behavioral patterns
Human and material resources*

The A.N.A. standards are written according to a systematic framework, the nursing process. They include continuously and systematically collecting data, which is recorded, kept accessible, and communicated. From this data base is derived a diagnosis. The diagnosis is then used to set a goal, identify priorities of action, and plan nursing intervention. All of this is completed by the joint efforts of patient and nurse working together to maximize the patient's health potential. After they implement the plan, patient and nurse jointly evaluate progress towards the goal and utilize this evaluation to determine needed reassessment, reordering of priorities, new goals, and revised planning.[2]

If the nursing process is utilized in professional practice, then personal values and those of the A.N.A. are aligned. If the nurse makes decisions for the patient and excludes him from the process, then the nurse's values will be in conflict with those expressed by A.N.A.

The A.N.A.'s specific practice divisions have established specific standards of practice for each specialty area. The practice divisions have begun to implement voluntary testing and evaluation procedures which determine whether or not a nurse in that specific division is meeting and maintaining these standards. Nurses who participate in this clearly value establishing, proclaiming, and behaving in accordance with the specific standards of practice.

For example, the A.N.A.'s psychiatric-mental health nursing practice division describes fourteen standards. There are standards for utilizing a scientific knowledge base, for data collection, for utilizing the nursing process, and for a problem solving approach in care plans. Other standards include involving the patient in the nursing process and cooperating with interdisciplinary approaches, the accountability of the nurse for her own behavior, and her responsibility for continuing education, professional development, and leadership. For each standard, a rationale is given, justifying the need for that standard. This is followed by specific factors to assess in determining whether or not this standard has been met.[3]

INSTITUTIONAL VALUES

Most nurses work in institutional settings, either private or governmental. Such institutions are usually structured bureaucratically. The standards and regulations are in accordance with the institution's needs and values to be economical and efficient. The rules and standards include task division and repetition of tasks. The decision making and control structure are hierarchial.[4]

McDonnell and associates point out the likelihood that bureaucratic standards

*Copyright by the American Nurses Association. Reprinted with permission.

will conflict with the ideal professional standards learned in nursing education. The bureaucratic system values are efficiency and economy, standardization, and external supervision. Learned professional ideals are more likely to consist of complete individualized patient care based on innovative application of knowledge by an autonomous nurse with collegial relationships.[4]

The opportunity for conflict is evident. Whenever innovative individualized patient care requires extra time, this value is in conflict with the bureaucratic value of efficiency and economy. The nurse who values automony may be in conflict with the bureaucratic value of external supervision.

Conflict with bureaucratic values may occur while the nurse is still a student. Student questions and requests of staff take time and may interfere with the efficiency of staff members. The priority of the clinical setting is to provide service, while the priority of those involved in education is learning. These differing priorities of staff and students suggest that conflict will occur.

Value conflict occurs both within personal values, and between personal values and professional values. Furthermore, value conflicts occur between professional and bureaucratic values and among professional, educational, and bureaucratic values. Any of these values has the potential to conflict with personal values.

EXPERIENCING VALUE CONFLICT

When value conflict occurs discomfort is experienced. An impending decision that involves values which are in opposition to one another will arouse uncomfortable feelings, bodily responses, and thoughts and will affect behavior. Personal discomfort may be the first indication of value conflicts. The conflict creates feelings of anxiety and ambivalence. The individual is likely to feel restless, unsettled, and uneasy; dread and/or fear may also be felt. Bodily responses may include: perspiration, muscle tension and aches, cold hands and feet, dry mouth, and nausea. In addition, the heart rate may increase and deep-sighing respiration may occur.

The experience of anxiety makes clear thinking more difficult. Ambivalent thoughts lead to doubt, indecision, and anxiety. Small amounts of anxiety increase attention and alertness but larger amounts of anxiety interfere with concentration and logical thinking. The thought process may be out of focus as if the individual were dazed after a blow to the head. Thoughts may jump around despite efforts to concentrate, or the individual may remain preoccupied with the problem but be unable to consider alternatives and consequences. Another possibility is ignoring the decision and its attendant problems, which can be done with or without awareness. If one is unaware of blocking the decision from awareness, feelings and behavior will be usual until something interferes with denial and repression. When awareness of the decision occurs, the discomfort will return in a rush.

Behavior reflects feelings and thoughts. Hesitant behavior, with tentative movement in one direction, reflects one value. When awareness of the opposing value occurs, behavior may turn to the other direction. Behavior may be very inconsistent as the individual behaves one way one hour and the opposite way the next hour. Inconsistency is also reflected in saying one thing and doing another. The individual may be unaware of this vacillating behavior. Observers may be more aware of the inconsistency than the behaving person.

Other behaviors which may indicate value conflict are automatic behaviors and immobilization; both are responses to high anxiety. In a routine situation a nurse may respond automatically, like a robot, out of touch with feelings and thoughts. If the nurse feels strongly pulled in two directions, inaction may result. The vacillation may be so strong that no inclination is enacted. This immobilization may be limited to the area involving the decision or it may spread to affect other behaviors.

All people have usual ways in which they cope with anxiety and problems. Behavior which occurs in the presence of value conflicts will likely be similar to behavior when experiencing other conflicts and anxiety. Usual patterns of coping may be moving out and against the source of discomfort; if this is the case, angry, demanding, and volatile behaviors will be seen. If one usually withdraws, shying away from problems, then this will be evident in behavior when value conflicts occur.

Several factors influence the degree of discomfort experienced with value conflicts. There will be greater discomfort if the values are strong values which are very important and if the discrepancy between the values involved is large. If the decision is very important and has long-lasting effects, discomfort will be increased. The length of time during which the conflict is experienced will also have an effect. Conflicts which occur and are resolved in an hour will have less effect than conflicts which persist over days, weeks, or months. Other life stress, usual coping style, and the presence of other people who are supportive and can help with problem solving will also affect the degree of discomfort.

RESOLVING VALUE CONFLICT

When discomfort is experienced, feelings, bodily responses, thoughts, and behaviors reflecting value conflict are identified; the nurse will want to resolve this conflict to facilitate making the decision. The resolution of the conflict will be based on values. It is necessary to identify and list the values involved on each side of the conflict. When lists of values involved are completed, an integration of the values into one rank-ordered list is needed. This rank ordering of values will strengthen some of the response possibilities and weaken others. This will decrease the conflict since the opposing directions will no longer be equally strong.

Identifying and rank ordering values is a difficult process. However, it adds a concrete and specific dimension and allows continuation with the components of this decision making process.

From studying the rank-ordered list of values, a strong value for a situation which is not listed may be discovered. The addition of this new value may introduce a new alternative for behavior which is more valued than either of the possibilities involved in the original conflict.

There may be ways of combining two values and therefore diminishing their conflicts. When differing values are combined into one list, there is the opportunity for an integration of previously conflicting values. McDonnell and co-workers compared the values of nurses identified by their nursing directors as being highly successful, average in success, or less than average in success in nursing. They found that both highly successful and minimally successful nurses held more educationally ideal professional values than average successful nurses. However, highly successful nurses also held more bureaucratic values, indicating that they had successfully integrated the two sets of values.[4]

SUMMARY

The existence of personal values, professional values, and bureaucratic values creates the ongoing probability of value conflict. Personal values reflect unique beliefs and experiences. Professional values, as stated by professional organizations, reflect ideals for action by members of the profession. Bureaucratic values usually involve efficiency and economy for the maintenance of the institution. It is not possible to avoid value conflicts because congruence is difficult with these three distinct sets of values.

It is possible to understand these different sets of values and to recognize value conflict when it occurs. Personal response to this conflict will most likely be discomfort. Anxious and ambivalent feelings may occur and thought processes may change. Behavior may be inconsistent, automatic, or immobilized. Coping adaptively with value conflict includes recognizing the problem, identifying the values involved, and putting these in priority. This will identify what is most important. This integrated list of priorities may also suggest ways to combine values or it may reveal omitted values. Recognition of personal priorities will be the guide to action.

EXAMPLE: Mary and Mark

This example utilizes the theory you have just read to demonstrate possible value conflicts which you might experience.

> Mary is junior student nurse. It is her second day in the psychiatric–mental health nursing rotation. Yesterday, Mary introduced herself to Mark and began to establish a therapeutic relationship. Mary told Mark who she was and why she was there, and said she would like to spend time with him learning to understand him from his point of view. She told him the days and times she would be available. They discussed confidentiality and Mark asked several questions as if to reasure himself that confidentiality really would exist.
>
> Today Mary found Mark in the lounge and asked if she could sit next to him. He nodded and said "Yes," as Mary sat down, Mark yawned. "Sleepy?" Mary said.

"Mmmmm," Mark responded. As Mary looked more closely at Mark, he leaned toward her and said, "Don't tell anyone, OK?" "OK," said Mary. Mark began, "My roommate has some really good grass last night so we went outside and got loaded. Just as we were about to come in, our other roommate came up with a bottle of vodka. We had another joint, then brought the bottle in to our room. We drank most of the night. I'm still really ripped."

As Mark finished talking, his team nurse came by with the medicine cart. She handed Mark his medicine, which he swallowed.

It took a moment before Mary felt the impact of what she heard and saw. Then she realized that drugs, alcohol, and medications should not be combined. She recalled reading last night about the ill effects of combining phenothiazines and alcohol. She simultaneously experienced the desire to say something about what she saw and heard and the desire to remain quiet.

Mary felt her heart begin to pound and perspiration crept across her body. She opened her mouth to speak and nothing came out. The patient had swallowed the medication and the nurse had moved on. In Mary's imagination she saw Mark sprawled on the floor convulsing or dying. Her next thought was of his glaring at her angrily saying, "Get away from me, you betrayed my trust."

"Where is my instructor?" Mary thought. Then she got up to look for her.

In this example, Mary experiences discomfort as soon as she realizes her conflict between wanting to say something and wanting to keep quiet. She has a conflict between assuring patient safety and physical integrity, and building and maintaining a trusting relationship. All of her nursing education has emphasized the former. The hospital emphasizes the former. Mary has read that building and maintaining a trusting relationship will be the basis of her learning experience in psychiatric–mental health nursing. Her instructor has said that physical needs are not the primary focus of this rotation and that her own learning is most important. Mary is not sure if this is a conflict between service institution and educational values. She is sure there is a conflict in her own values.

Mary's feelings include ambivalence and anxiety. There is also fear as she fantasizes possible outcomes. Bodily responses include tachycardia and perspiration. Her thought process is first clouded, then preoccupied with the problem. Her initial behavior is immobilization, following by her most usual student coping behavior of seeking help from her instructor. The discomfort is intensified by the divergence of the values and the possibility of a severe consequence involving physical danger, perhaps even death.

In a brief discussion with her instructor, Mary is quickly able to identify that her values underlying the desire to speak to the staff nurse were providing for physical safety and maintaining life. Her values underlying her desire to say nothing were keeping to herself something said in confidence and maintaining a trusting relationship. She rank orders these four values for herself as:

1. Maintaing life
2. Providing for physical safety

3. Maintaining a confidence
4. Building a trusting relationship

The succeeding steps in Mary's decision process will be discussed in the next chapters.

ACTIVITIES

These activities are designed to help you (1) meet the objectives of this chapter, and (2) practice utilizing your knowledge of value conflict.

ACTIVITY 1

a. List values held by the nursing profession and by bureaucratic systems.

Professional nursing values	*Bureaucratic system value*
1.	1.
2.	2.
3.	3.
4.	4.
5.	5.
6.	6.
7.	7.
8.	8.

b. Underline those bureaucratic system values held by your own institutional environment. Add to this list any additional values of your institutional environment.
c. Circle values from the two lists which conflict.
d. Star values from both lists which conflict with your own personal values. Write in the conflicting personal values.
e. Discuss the probability of conflicts among professional, institutional, and personal values for you and describe the conflicts most likely to occur.

ACTIVITY 2

a. List possible responses to value conflict.

Feelings	Bodily responses	Thoughts	Actions
1.	1.	1.	1.
2.	2.	2.	2.
3.	3.	3.	3.
4.	4.	4.	4.
5.	5.	5.	5.

b. Circle those responses which you believe are typical of you, then discuss your own pattern of response to values conflicts.

c. Discuss possible ways to resolve value conflict and describe those ways which are most typical of you.

ACTIVITY 3: Timmy: a pediatric patient

   You are caring for 6-year-old Timmy, who had surgery 5 days ago. He has had several complications and his life now seems to hang by a thin thread. You have cared for Timmy since before his surgery and know it is important to his recovery to encourage him and his will to live.

   This evening Timmy says to you "Mom says John (9-year-old idolized brother) came with her tonight. He's downstairs in the lobby. I want to see him so much. I know he's not allowed to visit but please sneak him up here for just a few minutes."

Complete the following activities for this situation:

a. List the professional, institutional, and personal values involved.

Professional	Institutional	Personal
1.	1.	1.
2.	2.	2.
3.	3.	3.

b. Rank order the values in each list for yourself.

Professional	Institutional	Personal
1.	1.	1.
2.	2.	2.
3.	3.	3.

c. Analyze the extent to which these values are your values by starring those values which you have freely chosen from other possibilities after consideration of the consequences of each. Underline those values which you cherish and publicly affirm. Circle those values which you act upon repeatedly and consistently.

d. Using your analysis for c as your guide, make one rank-ordered list of values from the three lists in b.

1.

2.

3.

4.

5.

6.

7.

8.

9.

e. Add any values which you can now see are missing from your list.

ACTIVITY 4: Fran: critical-care dilemma

You are working in critical care. Three days ago the head nurse called a staff meeting because the narcotic count had been off twice in the past 10 days. She asked all staff to be observant in the coming days for any irregularities or unexplained situations.

Today you are covering your friend Fran's patients, Mrs. Blue and Miss Snow, while Fran is at lunch. Fran said before she left that neither of them should need anything while she is gone. You stop by Mrs. Blue's bedside to check on her. She complains of pain and asks for medication. You check her chart and see that Fran has recorded meperidine (Demerol), 50 mg. IM, less than an hour ago. Mrs. Blue says she has not received a pain shot since breakfast. Puzzled, you go on to check Miss Snow and, with an uncomfortable sense of deja vu, you have almost the same experience with her. Miss Snow is insistent that she last had pain medication before breakfast, although Fran has recorded giving Demerol within the hour.

Complete the following activities for this situation.
a. List the professional, institutional, and personal values involved.

Professional	Institutional	Personal
1.	1.	1.
2.	2.	2.
3.	3.	3.

b. Rank order the values in each list for yourself.

Professional	Institutional	Personal
1.	1.	1.
2.	2.	2.
3.	3.	3.

c. Analyze the extent to which these values are your values by starring those values which you have freely chosen from other possibilities after consideration of the consequence of each. Underline those values which you cherish and publicly affirm. Circle those values which you act upon repeatedly and consistently.

d. Using your analysis from c as your guide, make one rank-ordered list of values from the three lists in b:
1.

2.

3.

4.

5.

6.

7.

8.

9.

e. Add any values which you can now see are missing from your list.

REFERENCES

1. National League for Nursing, Subcommittee on Records, June, 1957. Footnoted in Beland, I. L., and Matheney, R. V.: Patient-centered approaches to nursing, New York, 1960, The Macmillan Co.
2. Congress for Nursing Practice: Standards of nursing practice, Kansas City, 1973, American Nurses Association.
3. Congress for Nursing Practice: Standards of psychiatric-mental health nursing, Kansas City, 1973, American Nurses Association.
4. McDonnell, C., Kramer, M., and Leak, A.: What would you do? Am. J. Nurs. **72:**297, 1972.

5 DEVELOPING OBJECTIVES FROM VALUES

**BEHAVIORAL
OBJECTIVES**

After completing the activities in this chapter, you will be able to:

■ Discuss the relationship of behavioral objectives and values clarification in the decision making process.
■ Define the term "behavioral objective."
■ Identify and briefly discuss the components of general and specific behavioral objectives.
■ Discuss the differences between general and specific behavioral objectives.
■ Describe and briefly discuss the three major domains of behavioral objectives.
■ Given a situation in which values have been clearly stated, formulate complete behavioral objectives.
■ Discuss the relationship of behavioral objectives to the decision making process

In this chapter behavioral objectives are defined and related to values and the valuing process. The components and types of behavioral objectives are described, their function in the decision making process is discussed, and utilization is demonstated.

Value indicators suggest a behavioral direction which must be chosen freely with awareness of consequences, prized privately and publicly, and acted upon consistently to become an actualized value.

Clearly stated, actualized values are behavioral statements. They describe a consistent behavior or attitude which has evolved from choosing and prizing. Behavioral objectives describe the action to be exhibited as a result of values held;

they are guidelines for initiating and maintaining action. Behavioral objectives may be utilized in the latter part of the valuing process to plan implementation of the consistent behavior or they may be used with fully actualized values to plan the continued specific and consistent implementation of such values. Either way, the behavioral objectives are clearly stated plans for action.

COMPONENTS OF BEHAVIORAL OBJECTIVES

Writing a behavioral objective is writing a plan for the continued enactment of a value. Both clearly stated values and behavioral objectives contain a subject and object reference and an action verb. The subject and object references and action verb answer the question, "Who does what?" In the example in Chapter 3, Jeanine values eating natural food. Jeanine is the subject reference, natural food is the object reference, and eating is the action verb. Jeanine is the "who," eating the "does," and natural foods the "what." "Jeanine values eating natural food" is a clearly stated value, while "Jeanine will eat natural food" is a behavioral objective describing the implementation of the value.

The action verb of the behavioral objective is the key guideline; it tells what will be done. This verb must be carefully chosen to reflect doing something which is in some way observable. Directly observable performances are more easily acknowledged than indirectly observable performances. When unobservable performances are desired, an observable indicator must be given. For example, if the desired performance is valuing or preferring natural foods, an observable indicator such as choosing or eating is stated.

Two types of behavioral objectives may be written: general and specific. A *general* objective contains subject and object references and an action verb which answers the question, "Who will do what?" In addition to subject and object references and an action verb, a *specific* behavioral objective contains criteria for measurement from which evaluation of attainment of the behavioral objective is possible. Specific evaluation criteria indicate the conditions under which the behavior is to occur and the extent or level of accomplishment which is expected. Evaluation criteria answer the questions where, when, and how well or to what extent.

If two individuals saw Jeanine eating an apple, they would likely agree that Jeanine was fulfilling her objective to eat natural foods. If the same two individuals observed Jeanine eating an apple and processed cheese, they might disagree as to whether or not she was implementing her value. Must she always eat only natural foods, or does acting according to the value mean eating natural foods when they are available, or 80 percent of the time, or two out of three meals? Any of these is a possible criterion for measurement. Under what conditions must she eat natural foods? At home? At home and at friends' homes? At all times? These conditions are also evaluation criteria. In specific behavioral objectives, these criteria are stated.

Specific behavioral objectives are useful because the evaluation criteria is specific and, at any given time, it is possible to determine whether or not the objective is fulfilled. If Jeanine's objective is to eat natural foods 50 percent of the time wherever she may be, it is obvious that she is fulfilling the objective of half of her lunch is natural food. If her objective is to eat natural foods 80 percent of the time wherever she may be, then information about breakfast and dinner is needed to determine whether or not she fulfills the objective (behaves according to the value). These specific evaluation criteria are not contained in clear statements of a value or general objectives ("Jeanine values natural foods," or "Jeanine will eat natural foods"). They are stated in specific behavioral objectives such as, "Jeanine will eat natural foods 50 percent of the time wherever she may be."

In this example, "50 percent of the time" answers the question how well or to what extent Jeanine will eat natural foods. "Wherever she may be" specifies the conditions under which Jeanine will eat natural foods. Both the conditions and the performance criteria (how well or to what extent) are essential for a specific behavioral objective.

In the example in Chapter 2, Bill's behavior reflects his value of giving emotional support. The implied general behavioral objective can be written for Bill based on his behavior within the context: "I will give emotional support." Bill is the subject reference, emotional support is the object reference, and giving is the action verb. Bill is the "who," giving is the "does," and emotional support is the "what."

Bill's place of employment and behavior reflect the conditions. The emergency room is "where" Bill gives emotional support, and after delegating essential tasks, assessing and intervening in life-threatening situations is "when" support is given. Another condition, evident from Bill's behavior within the context, is giving support freely rather than in response to external requests or overt stimuli. This is the performance criterion, or "extent" to which he will offer support. In this situation. Bill's behavior may be the fulfillment of his own specific behavioral objective: "While working in the emergency room, I will freely offer emotional support to patients after delegating essential tasks and assessing and intervening in life-threatening situations."

Behavioral objectives have been developed primarily as communication in the teaching-learning process. The developer of an educational experience writes the specific behaviors which the student is expected to achieve from given circumstances and experiences. The behaviors and evaluation criteria need to be very exacting so that the student is clear as to what must be done.

When objectives are written for personal use, the evaluation criteria may or may not need to be as specific as for learning objectives. There is disagreement among professionals as to whether evaluation criteria should be general or detailed and specific. This question is pertinent for the personal use of behavioral objectives. Specific behavioral objectives are easier to measure because of their specific evaluation criteria, but often they are more difficult to write. Sometimes only general objectives are appropriate for the situation. Both can be useful. The important point is that the objectives are clear to you since they will be your reference point in identifying problems and continuing with the decision making process.

DOMAINS OF BEHAVIORAL OBJECTIVES

Behavioral objectives may be written in any of the three domains of learning and performance: cognitive, affective, and psychomotor. The cognitive domain is concerned with knowledge and thinking, the affective domain reflects feelings and emotions, while the psychomotor domain is the physical, muscular enactment of mental processes. Although these domains are discussed separately, they are interrelated and interdependent in their development and implementation.

The behaviors in all three domains may be arranged in a developmental progression called a taxonomy. Various authors have composed such taxonomies. Reilly[1] is particularly helpful to the nursing profession because she has applied three taxonomies to the nursing educational situation.

Bloom and associates[2] arranged cognitive objectives into a simple to complex progression beginning with recall and progressing to synthesis and evaluation: the levels are knowledge, comprehension, application, analysis, synthesis, and evaluation. Knowledge is the recall of information, from isolated facts to complex theories. With comprehension one understands a situation, from grasping some aspects to comprehending all the possible implications of a situation. This may be demonstrated simply by giving an illustration or more complexly by explanation or the prediction of consequences. Application refers to the utilization of knowledge in real situations. Analysis requires the identification and understanding of component parts and their relationship to each other and to the whole structure. Synthesis is the joining of parts into a whole structure which is new to the participant. Evaluation requires judgment to determine worth according to internal and/or external guidelines.

"Given a written quiz, Jeanine will list five natural foods" is a specific behavioral objective requiring the recall of isolated facts. An example of complex information which is still at the recall level of knowledge is "When given an examination in class, Jeanine will describe with 95 percent accuracy three theories which may be used to interpret the role of additives and preservatives in promoting or diminishing health." At the complex end of the spectrum are examples of synthesis and evaluation: "Within three days Jeanine will propose to the class a dietary plan for improving her health through increasing by 50 percent her intake of natural vitamin C," and "Jeanine will simultaneously evaluate her proposed plan according to three published research studies of natural foods."

A taxonomy of objectives for the development of behaviors in the affective domain was devised by Krathwohl and co-workers.[3] The developmental progression in this domain is toward personal growth with the evolution of a personal value system which becomes the basis for congruent behavior. The identified steps are receiving, responding, valuing, organizing, and characterizing by a value or value complex. The three steps of receiving are awareness, willingness to receive, and attention to specific stimuli. Awareness is the conscious recognition of a particular situation. With willingness to receive, one desires this conscious recognition and observes without judgment or avoidance, first to total situations then to selected aspects of those situations.

Responding may first be from/to external expectations; with development, it stems from internal expectations and is accompanied by emotional satisfaction. Valuing is the process discussed in Chapter 3: belief or the attachment of worth is chosen freely from alternatives with awareness of consequences, prized publicly and privately, and acted upon consistently. Organization occurs when the interrelationship of values is recognized and conceptualized and priorities are established. In characterization by a value or value complex, the individual achieves extensive congruence between values and behavior. An internally consistent, integrated value system is repeatedly reflected in multiple behavior patterns. There is a strong interelationship between cognitive and affective processes.

Bill's behavior reflects the development of behaviors in the affective domain. Bill recognizes a situation where emotional support is ususally needed (receiving through awareness) and responds supportively because he values this response in himself and feels good about responding this way. He demonstrates an integrated system of values. Bill values giving emotional support and also values the maintenance of life. When only one of these values can be expressed behaviorally at one time, Bill first enacts life-maintaining behaviors. He understands the interdependence of values on one another and believes he can foster both best by maintaining life first, then providing emotional support to enhance the quality of life.

Through a developmental progression of coordination, Dave[4] describes a taxonomy of psychomotor domain behaviors. The range is imitation, manipulation, precision, articulation, and naturalization. Imitation, the learning of motor skills by observation, is followed by manipulation, performing motor skills. With further progression, precision becomes more exact and independent until movement is a harmonious sequence of behaviors (articulation). With the highest coordination of psychomotor behaviors, single skillful acts are performed both automatically and spontaneously as a means to an end which is an integration of cognitive, affective, and psychomotor behavior.

Bill's behavior in assessing and intervening in life-threatening behavior must include a number of motor skills that have been learned and developed into precise acts, which are part of his harmonious sequence of assessment skills. Bill performs these skills automatically as he attends to the patient for the promotion, restoration, or maintenance of health.

Components of a specific behavioral objective

Subject reference (who)	Action verb (will do)	Object reference (what)	Under what conditions (where, when)	To what extent (how well)

Behavioral domains

Cognitive (thinking)	Affective (feelings, attitudes)	Psychomotor (skills)
↓	↓	↓
Knowledge	Receipt	Imitation
↓	↓	↓
Comprehension	Response	Manipulation
↓	↓	↓
Application	Valuing	Precision
↓	↓	↓
Analysis	Organization	Articulation
↓	↓	↓
Synthesis	Characterization	Naturalization
↓		
Evaluation		

After values are clarified, behavioral objectives help to integrate the domains of learning and performance. This integration of domains is essential for personally congruent, effective decision making. Intellectual skills are applied to the affective domain of valuing to determine congruent psychomotor application. Specific objectives then facilitate the translation of values into behavior by describing the behavior which will demonstrate the value.

Cognitive objectives at the knowledge and comprehension level are the easiest to measure. It is simple to determine if terms have been defined, components have been listed, or an example has been given. Objectives for cognitive evaluation, affective characterization, or psychomotor skill naturalization are inherently more difficult to measure because of their complexity.

SUMMARY

Behavioral objectives are the guidelines for action in translating values into behavior. General and specific objectives contain a subject and object reference and action verb which answer the question: "Who does what?" Specific objectives also describe the conditions under which the behavior is to occur and the level of performance to be achieved. These evaluation criteria answer the questions "Where, when, and how well or to what extent?"

Behavioral objectives may be written in the cognitive, affective, or psychomotor domains of learning. Cognitive objectives are for intellectual achievement, affective objectives are for the development of feelings, attitudes, and values, and psychomotor objectives are for motor skill development. Personally congruent, effective decision making depends on an integration of these domains.

EXAMPLE 1: Mr. Jones

This example demonstrates behavioral objectives written in all three domains.

Mr. Jones, age 39, is a recently diagnosed hypertensive patient. As a result of a community screening clinic, his blood pressure was found to be markedly elevated, he was referred to a physician for diagnostic work-up and evaluation. Based on the information and data obtained, Mr. Jones was started on antihypertensive drug therapy and referred to the nurse practitioner within the physician's office for education and follow-up. Mr. Jones has attended several teaching sessions with the practitioner and they discussed the life-style alterations of (1) diet—low sodium, low cholesterol, and calorie restriction; (2) reduction of stress and tension; (3) weight reduction; (4) cessation of smoking; and (5) regular and consistent exercise. Drug side effects and self-measurement of blood pressure were taught to him. Based on these educational sessions, Mr. Jones has written the following general objectives for himself.

COGNITIVE OBJECTIVES

Comprehension To recognize "correct and appropriate" sounds when performing self-measurement of blood pressure.
Application To plan a balanced daily diet which is low in sodium, cholesterol, and calories, having been given a general knowledge of nutrition.
Analysis To identify those factors which cause emotional stress and tension.
Synthesis To interpret to others the feelings experienced as a result of overwhelming life-style changes and the diagnosis of a chronic illness.
Evaluation To assess health care in terms of completeness, satisfaction, and results.

AFFECTIVE OBJECTIVES

Receiving To be aware of the available community resources for hypertensive screening and for hypertensive patients and their families.
Responding To cooperate with the exercise and weight reduction programs.
Valuing To accept the life-style changes that accompany the diagnosis of hypertension.
Organization To relate to and interact with others in a manner consistent with the rehabilitation goal of decreased tension, stress, and anxiety.
Characterization To develop a code of general behavior consistent with maintenance and preservation of health.

PSYCHOMOTOR OBJECTIVES

Imitation To perform self-measurement of blood pressure after observing a demonstration of the procedure.
Manipulation To demonstrate correct placement of the sphygmomanometer and stethoscope.
Precision To recognize the difference between systolic and diastolic blood pressure sounds.
Articulation To measure blood pressure within one minute accurately.
Naturalization To measure blood pressure with the results corresponding to within ± 5 min. Hg of results obtained by an experienced health professional.[5]

EXAMPLE 2: Mary and Mark

This example demonstrates behavioral objectives derived directly from values.

Review the example from Chapter 4, "Mary and Mark." Mary has ranked her values as:

1. Maintaining life
2. Providing for physical safety
3. Maintaining a confidence

Mary writes the following specific behavioral objectives to implement her values:

1. When providing patient care I will consistently perform nursing functions that promote the maintenance of life.
2. When providing patient care, I will continuously assess and provide for physical safety.
3. When providing patient care, I will always maintain patient confidences.

In objective 1, "Mary" is the "who" (subject reference), "will perform" is the "does" (action verb), and "nursing functions" is the "what" (object reference). "When giving patient care" describes the conditions of "when" and "where" this behavior will take place. "Consistently" describes "how well" or "to what extent" the life-maintaining actions will be implemented.

In objective 2, Mary is the "who," assess and provide the "doing," and physical safety the "what." "When providing patient care" descirbes the conditions of "when" and "where" this behavior will take place, "continuously" describes the "extent" of assessing and providing for physical safety.

In objective 3, Mary is the "who," "will maintain" is thc "docs," and "patient confidences" is the "what." As in objectives 1 and 2, "when providing patient care" describes the conditions of "when" and "where" the behavior is to occur. "Always" describes the extent to which patient confidences will be maintained.

ACTIVITIES

These activities are designed to help you review the content of the chapter to meet the objectives.

ACTIVITY 1

Define the term "behavioral objective."

ACTIVITY 2

Identify the five essential components of a specific behavioral objective and state the questions answered by each of these components.

ACTIVITY 3

After reading the following objectives, identify those which are not specific behavioral objectives and make them so.

a. I will write behavioral objectives for myself.

b. Given a list of possible job values, I will rank the values for myself and translate three into behavioral objectives.

c. Given a situation involving value conflicts, I will resolve the conflict.

ACTIVITY 4

Discuss the relationship of behavioral objectives to values and to the decision making process as a whole.

These activities are designed to provide practice in utilizing behavior objectives as a component of the decision making process.

ACTIVITY 5

Read the following situation and complete the exercises.

Mrs. Mills is the Continuing Education Coordinator for the local community hospital; she provides continuing education classes for hospital employees. A recent baccalaureate graduate from the local university, her nursing curriculum was learning and teaching based upon behavioral objectives. A firm believer in this type of learning, she prepares her continuing education classes on the basis of behavioral objectives. She has just completed cardiopulmonary resuscitation (CPR) classes for all hospital personnel. Her primary aim for the CPR classes was to provide all hospital personnel with the ability to assess respiratory or cardiac arrest, initiating and maintaining CPR according to Heart Association standards wherever and whenever called upon to do so.

a. Identify Mrs. Mills' values.

b. Write a behavioral objective reflecting Mrs. Mills' value of continuing education.

c. In terms of Mrs. Mills' values for continuing education, write one objective reflective of each of the following categories:
    1. Cognitive domain

    2. Affective domain

    3. Psychomotor domain

d. Write a CPR behavioral objective for the following:
    1. Beginning nursing student

    2. Senior nursing student

    3. Nurse practitioner (or clinician)

e. Do you think Mrs. Mills' behavioral objectives would vary with the knowledge base of the individuals she was teaching; e.g., physicians, nurses, housekeeping personnel, dietary personnel? If so, why?

f. How does the primary aim for the class as stated by Mrs. Mills meet the criteria for a specific behavioral objective so as to meet her value of continuing education?[5]

ACTIVITY 6

From the following list of possible job values, select ten which are most important to you and rank them in order of importance. Write behavioral objectives from at least the five most important values. Look at the list of job possibilities and decide which job possibility might best fulfill the behavioral objectives.

POSSIBLE JOB VALUES

Variety
Security
Authority
Prestige
High salary
Talking with people
Location
Doing research
Working with a team of people
Technical expertise
Applying the latest
  scientific knowledge
Independence
Access to continuing education
Consultation availability
Minimal physical activity
Daytime hours
Weekday hours
Opportunity to travel
Working with the aged
Working with women
Working with children

Excellent supervision
Minimal interactional
  requirements
Intellectual stimulation
Emotional satisfaction
Challenge
Multiple decisions to make
Wear a uniform
Administrative
  responsibilities
No administrative
  responsibilities
Clinical expertise
Clinical judgment required
Clients similar to me
Clients different from me
Teaching students
Teaching patients
No teaching responsibilities
No nursing care
Working alone
Other

BEHAVIORAL OBJECTIVES

1.

2.

3.

4.

5.

JOB POSSIBILITIES

Job	*Area*	
Staff nurse	Pediatrics	
Team leader	Obstetrics	In hospital
Head nurse	Gynecology	clinic or day
Supervisor	Medicine	treatment center
Clinical specialist	Surgery	
Administrator	Psychiatry	
Practitioner	Rehabilitation	
Teacher	ICU	
Consultant	CCU	
Researcher	ER	
	Operating Room	
	Public health	
	Industry	
	Community mental health center	
	Womens' health care center	
	Free clinic	
	Licensed Vocational Nurse	
	Community college	
	University program	
	Graduate program	
	American Nurses Association	
	State planning agency	
	School nurse	

ACTIVITY 7: Timmy: a pediatric patient

You are caring for 6-year-old Timmy, who had surgery 5 days ago. He has had several complications and his life now seems to hang by a thin thread. You have cared for Timmy since before his surgery and know it is important to his recovery to encourage him and his will to live.

This evening Timmy says to you, "Mom says John (9-year-old idolized brother) came with her tonight. He's downstairs in the lobby. I want to see him so much. I know he's not allowed to visit but please sneak him up here for just a few minutes."

In the activities in Chapter 4 you have already ranked your values for this situation. Rewrite the three most important values here:

1.

2.

3.

Your task for this chapter is to write three specific behavioral objectives to implement each of these values.

1.

2.

3.

Do your objectives have a subject and object reference and an action verb indicating "Who will do what?" Have you specified under what conditions and to what extent this behavior will take place? Does this answer "Where, when, and how well?" Will you and/or an observer know when the objective has been fulfilled?

ACTIVITY 8: Fran: critical-care dilemma

You are working in critical care. Three days ago the head nurse called a staff meeting because the narcotic count had been off twice in the past 10 days. She asked all staff to be observant in the coming days for any irregularities or unexplained situations.

Today you are covering your friend Fran's patients, Mrs. Blue and Miss Snow, while Fran is at lunch. Fran said before she left that neither of them should need anything while she is gone. You stop by Mrs. Blue's bedside to check on her. She complains of pain and asks for medication. You check her chart and see that Fran has recorded meperidine (Demerol), 50 mg. IM, less than an hour ago. Mrs. Blue says she has not received a pain shot since breakfast. Puzzled, you go on to check Miss Snow and, with an uncomfortable sense of deja vu, you have almost the same experience with her. Miss Snow is insistent that she last had pain medication before breakfast, although Fran has recorded giving Demerol within the hour.

In Chapter 4 you have already rank-ordered your values for this situation. Rewrite the three most important values here:

1.

2.

3.

Your task in this chapter is to write three specific behavioral objectives to implement each of these values.

1.

2.

3.

Does your objective have a subject and object reference and an action verb indicating "Who will do what?" Have you specified under what conditions and to what extent this behavior will take place? Does this answer "Where, when, and how well?" Will you and/or an observer know when the objective has been fulfilled?

REFERENCES

1. Reilly, D. E.: Behavioral objectives in nursing: evaluation of learner attainment, New York, 1975, Appleton-Century-Crofts.
2. Bloom, B. S., editor: Taxonomy of educational objectives: the classification of educational goals. Handbook I: cognitive domain, New York, 1956, David McKay Co., Inc.
3. Krathwohl, D. R., Bloom, B. S., and Masia, B. B.: Taxonomy of educational objectives: the classification of educational goals. Handbook II: Affective domain, New York, 1968, David McKay Co., Inc.
4. Dave, R. H. Quoted in Reilly, D. E.: Behavioral objectives in nursing. New York, 1975, Appleton-Century-Crofts.
5. Cleveland, L.: Unpublished manuscript, 1977.

6 IDENTIFYING PROBLEMS

BEHAVIORAL OBJECTIVES

After completing the activities in this chapter, you will be able to:

- Discuss the relationship of problem identification to behavioral objectives and values.
- Define the term "problem" as utilized in this decision making process.
- Discuss how knowledge, skill, past experience, and situational characteristics influence problem identification.
- Discuss the formulation of a problem statement from a problem area.
- Make a concise problem statement from a general problem area.

Many people begin the problem solving or decision making process with recognition of a problem.[1-4] However, in the decision making process presented in this book, problem identification is part of the continuum of the process. Values clarification sets the framework for the decision making process. Values are clarified and from them behavioral objectives are developed. Once these aspects of the decision making process are learned and utilized, they become ongoing occurrences in one's life. Individuals continually behave according to their values; that is, they strive to fulfill the behavioral objectives they have set for themselves. All goes well if they consistently meet the behavioral objectives and thus operate by values they have ranked. This is the ideal state one strives for but rarely achieves on a daily basis. Behavioral objectives may not be met. This situation of unmet behavioral objectives results in a problem. A problem, as defined in this process, results from the nonachievement of a stated objective. A problem is a potential or actual threat to one's objectives and thus to one's value system.

This definition of a problem differs from definitions commonly found in the nursing literature.[2,5] Differentiation of patients' and nurses' problems are emphasized by the nursing profession. Certain patient needs and problems are commonly identified in various ways. For example, patient problems are defined as disturbances of the patient need system, a determination made by the nurse. Nursing problems are obstacles the nurse encounters in assisting the patient to meet these needs.[2] Such definitions are not in conflict with the use of "problem" presented here, but one should be aware of the differences in the use of the term when proceeding with this process.

Problems result from unmet or threatened objectives. These unmet or threatened objectives also threaten the value system as values are the basis for the objectives. Just as the definition of problem in this process differs from those frequently used in nursing education, so may the designated cause of problems vary. The differences, in actuality, are one of perspective. For example, one may value maintaining life. A patient's cardiac arrest threatens this value, resulting in a problem. This same situation, cardiac arrest, causes the patient to have physiological instability. He has a need for oxygen to his vital organs. The need for oxygen is unmet and a patient problem, as commonly defined, results. Thus the interpretation of the "problem" may differ but the basic reasoning behind the problem identification is similar.

The interpretation of "problem" as described in this process is broad. This view of a problem recognizes the fact that the definition of one's needs is based on one's values. There is no one set of needs agreed upon; if such a list did exist, identification of needs would still be subjective. For example, consider a dying patient who sees his problem as remaining alert as long as possible to be with his family; one nurse may see he needs physical comfort measures, and another nurse may think he needs emotional support. Each would attempt to meet the need, and thus the patient problem, in various ways. Problems which are defined only in terms of disturbed need areas are thus subjective. The definition used in this process recognizes that needs come from values, a more comprehensive approach. Acknowledgement is made of the fact that because values are different for each individual, so must needs and problems also vary.

IDENTIFICATION OF PROBLEM AREAS

The identification of problems may be either easy or difficult. Some problems are very obvious; others are vague or covert. The sources of problems are innumerable. Problems can arise from any part of one's environment, internal or external. Problems may arise from within oneself, physically or psychologically. For example, a broken leg may threaten one's value of being freely mobile, disease may threaten one's health values, loneliness may pose a threat to the value of being independent. In each of these situations the threat comes from one's internal being. External sources such as people, jobs, or money may also threaten one's values. Every day one faces a multitude of situations which may result in problems. Each person encounters different sets of stimuli, both internal and external. Any of these can result in a problem at that point in time if one's objectives and thus one's values are potentially or actually threatened.

INFORMATION GATHERING AND INTERPRETATION

Information gathering and interpretation are prerequisite to problem recognition. Information is the basis for problem determination, as it is through information that an individual determines if a threat to his values exists. Information gathering is an ongoing process. One continually is monitoring the environment, both internal and external, for information. The sources of this data are numerous. Individuals rely on such bodily sensations as pain, hunger, and tactile input for internal data. Vision and hearing provide a great deal of information about the external environment. Television, books, movies, and other people constantly bring one information about the world. For nurses, too, the sources of information are broad. The patient himself is often the most important source for information, but families, relatives, and friends also provide data. Progress notes, Kardexes, laboratory reports, radiographic findings, end-of-the-shift report, and consultations with health care team members all give information. Information may be readily available or one may have to search diligently for it.

Information gathering requires an open mind, a state which facilitates decision making. Problems are not failures. Problems occur daily; they are a part of living, not always a result of an oversight or mistake. Seeing problems as failures often results in blaming either oneself or others. Blaming turns the focus of problems to the past. The past cannot be changed and frustration results.[6] By focusing on the present or future, problems can be identified and handled. Problems serve as challenges. One learns and grows from the decision making process.

Whatever the source or however easy or difficult the search for data, information gathering alone is not sufficient for problem recognition. Information must be interpreted. Data interpretation is essential for problem area identification. Interpretation of the information involves identification of what is known and what is needed. For example, as Joe White, R.N. is giving Ms. Caruthers her morning care he notices that her skin feels warm to the touch. Interpretation of this data includes information such as: she is third-day postoperative, her vital signs (last taken at 6:00 A.M.) were within normal limits, and Joe cared for her yesterday and her skin was cool. Joe decides he needs to take her temperature, check about any medication she is receiving, check on the results of wound culture taken yesterday, and check to see if IPPB has been ordered. The identification of what is known leads him to identify sources of information he does not know. This information is interpreted by Joe as he systematically explores a problem area. He does not yet know the precise problem but does recognize a general problem area that requires investigation. Warm skin is recognized as a deviation from normal. This occurrence threatens his value of promoting optimal recovery for his patients. His behavioral objective and value are threatened and a problem area is recognized.

How much information to gather and what sources of information to explore will be different for any given situation. In an emergency situation time may prohibit additional information gathering. At other times—for example, in making long-range discharge plans—more sources of information can be utilized. There are no set numbers or sources of information to use as a standard; this is situationally determined.

PROBLEM IDENTIFICATION

Knowledge, skill, past experience, and situational characteristics which influence one's perspective are several of the factors influencing problem identification. These factors influence problem recognition because they affect information gathering and interpretation of information.

Knowledge

One's knowledge base helps determine the type of information one seeks as well as the interpretation of the data. The more knowledge one has about a situation, the more precise the data gathering and interpretation can be. An individual with limited knowledge about certain factors may not see the existence of a problem area at all or may define the problem quite broadly. One with expertise in the area may be able to concisely state the problem using the knowledge one has to select and gather appropriate information. For example, consider a situation in a well-child clinic. Mrs. Becker brings in her 6-month-old, 24-pound baby girl. The aide, Jane Jackson, asks Mrs. Becker if there are any problems and how things are going. Mrs. Becker tells her everything is great—no problems at all. The aide notes the baby seems large and is unable to hold her head steadily. She reports this information to Sue Barnes, Pediatric Nurse Practitioner (PNP), telling her the baby seems delayed. Sue notes the baby's weight, checks the birth weight in the chart, and sees the child has gained 16 pounds since birth. The child has tripled her birth weight at 6 months; normally this takes a year. Sue gathers additional information such as careful diet history and developmental screening. From this information she defines the problem as: obese infant with secondary developmental delay. Each person's level of knowledge led to the interpretation of data. Mrs. Becker, the mother, sees no problem: the baby is gaining weight, causing no difficulties. Mrs. Jackson, the aide, knows something is not right: the child seems large and cannot hold her head. Mrs. Barnes, the PNP, is able to make a precise problem identification. This does not mean one person is right and another wrong. Each person used his own knowledge base to judge or scrutinize the information at hand. More information leads to more precise gathering, resulting in a higher-level interpretation. All used the same process but the results were different. Knowledge base is a major variable affecting the type of information sought, sources of information utilized, and interpretation of data.

Skill

Knowledge and skill may influence problem recognition in a similar manner. One's level of skill, the ability to do certain tasks, will influence problem identification. One may have knowledge about the mechanisms of blood pressure, but skill is required to perform the task. Thus skill adds important information to data interpretation. Knowledge and skill will vary among individual nurses. Different specialty areas are based on knowledge and skills inherent to that condition, age, or disease. A nurse who is a diabetes specialist will gather and interpret information about a new diabetic patient differently than a student who just read about diabetes mellitus for the first time last evening. Levels of knowledge and skill are important. Again, problem areas are not designated as right or wrong, but precision in problem identification is enhanced by one's knowledge and skill of the general problem area.

Past experience

Although knowledge and skill appear to influence problem recognition in a positive manner, past experience can have either a positive or negative influence. Past experience often colors information gathering and interpretation. One may jump ahead and make interpretations without fully assessing the situation. For example, Mr. Hanson works on an adolescent unit and has learned that peer visiting helps patients' morale and motivation toward recovery. One night, after seeing friends leave Susie Camp's room, he finds her crying. He knows visits provide a positive experience and thus discounts this influence and goes on looking for other possible sources of her distress. In actuality Susie has a Foley catheter and was frantic about her friends seeing it. Mr. Hanson's past experience became a negative influence.

Positive results from one's experience are possible. Past experience with a particular patient facing a certain stimulus may be very helpful. For example, Ms. Smith is caring for an asthmatic patient who suffers increased bronchoconstriction when her fluid intake is decreased. Dr. Jones has order Mrs. Graves to have nothing by mouth for 12 hours prior to laboratory tests. Ms. Smith carefully assesses Mrs. Graves regularly for early signs of breathing difficulties. She asked for an order to provide intravenous fluids if dyspnea occurs. Past experience has enabled Ms. Smith to better utilize information. Her assessment of information is precise, and she has developed a plan to deal with the potential problem.

Situational characteristics

The characteristics of a given situation influence one's information gathering and interpretations. Feeling states may alter this process. If one is anxious, tired, or fearful, the amount of information he receives may be limited in amount or scope. Time is another major factor. One may have to limit information gathering to a few details or one may be able to investigate a whole variety of information sources; time determines the scope. Availability of resources is also important. For example, one may be working alone with an unconscious patient and find that information resources are limited as a result of the situation.

Situational characteristics may influence one's perspective, which in turn affects information gathering and interpretation and thus problem recognition. One's perspective or outlook can determine the significance placed on certain cues or stimuli one encounters. For example, a nurse who works in an ambulatory psychiatric clinic may well know the symptoms of physical disease but her orientation to the psychosocial aspects of illness may interfere with her recognition of such problems. It is not that her knowledge base is inadequate, but her perspective influences her interpretation of data and therefore problem recognition.

•   •   •

Knowledge, skill, past experience, and situational characteristics are the factors that influence the manner in which one gathers information as well as the type of information sought or received. Data interpretation also depends on these factors. Clarifying values and developing behavioral objectives are not sufficient. One must constantly survey the environment for potential or actual threats so that appropriate action can be taken. For the decision making process to be effective, problems must be specifically identified.

NARROWING THE PROBLEM

A precise problem statement is the goal of this stage of the decision making process. This problem statement can be made if the general problem area is narrowed into a specific problem. Problems can be narrowed by determining the threat to the objective and thus to the value. Because a problem results from an *actual* or *potential* threat to one's objectives, two types of problems result: (1) one in which an aspect or aspects of the objective is/are not being met, and (2) one in which a potential threat to an objective occurs. Identification of the threat to the objective in either of these situations allows one to narrow the general problem area into a specific problem.

The use of specific behavioral objectives makes the first type of problem narrowing easy to accomplish. The aspect of the objective which is threatened is identified. For example, in some situations the "when" may be causing the objective to be unmet. Staff nurse Julie Lee's objective might be, "I will teach Mrs. Smith to give herself her first insulin injection today so she can independently give herself an injection tomorrow." At the end of the shift, she rushes in, harried, and gives Mrs. Smith the injection, telling herself, "I'll teach her tomorrow." This situation may become a problem for Julie. She may feel frustrated and angry. These feelings make her aware of a potential problem. Reflecting, she is able to identify the problem area—providing optimal care for Mrs. Smith. She can then narrow this general problem to a specific one. The "when" of the objective has not been fulfilled. Thus the problem becomes, "Today I was unable to teach Mrs. Smith to give herself the injection.

The "what" of the objective can also be unmet, leading to a problem area. For example, Janice James, a nurse, highly values the right of individuals to follow their cultural practices. Her objective for this value might be, "I will consistently encourage all patients to follow their cultural practices in meeting their health needs." One day as she cares for Mrs. Jimenez in the postpartum ward Janice finds her attempts to convince Mrs. Jimenez to breast feed are met with failure. All Janice's explanations are ignored. Mrs. Jimenez believes formula is better for her child; none of her friends or family feel breast feeding is right. Janice leaves frustrated and upset. She sees the general problem areas as "an uncooperative patient." Exploration of this situation enables Janice to see her objective has been unmet. The "what," encourage all patients to follow their cultural practices, has not been fulfilled and her value is threatened. The problem in this situation would be, "I did not encourage Mrs. Jimenez to follow her cultural practice regarding breast feeding."

Similar problems can be identified in situations in which the "who," "where," or "how well" of the objective is unmet. In some circumstances more than one component of the objective may be unmet; all of these components would be included in the problem.

Problem narrowing can also be accomplished with the second type of problem in which a potential threat to an objective exists. In some situations the objective may be currently met but is potentially threatened. Identification of the factors causing the threat narrows this type of problem. For example, Janice James had the objective, "I will consistently encourage all patients to follow their cultural practices in meeting their health needs." This objective may be threatened by the fact that there is a sudden increase in Vietnamese patients coming into Janice's unit, a culture about which Janice knows little. She cannot encourage her patients to follow their cultural practices if she does not know what these are. Her objective is potentially threatened. Her problem in this situation is, "I cannot encourage Vietnamese patients to follow their cultural practices."

Thus a problem is stated as a specific statement of the component of an objective which is not being currently met or a statement of the threat to an objective.

PROBLEM STATEMENT

This narrowing of the problem area leads to the formulation of a problem statement. The problem statement is in actuality a question which asks, "How can I maintain my value in this situation?" Thus Janice would next make a problem statement. She now looks at the potential threat to see how it can be managed. She must ask herself, "How can I encourage Vietnamese patients to follow their cultural practices in meeting their health needs?" This question is her problem statement.

The problem statement is the impetus for continuing with the decision making process. Not only must the specific problem be identified, but a search for resolution must be initiated. The problem statement serves this purpose. Problem statements must be objective; possible solutions are not part of a problem statement. The focus of the decision maker at this time is only the problem itself. Solutions proposed at this time do not allow for full analysis of the situation to select the best alternative possible. Objectivity in identifying the problem enables the decision maker to proceed with the process with an open mind.

SUMMARY

Problem identification is the impetus for the decision making process. The process of clarifying values and making behavioral objectives is ongoing. Awareness of a problem begins with a threatened value and thus an unfulfilled or threatened objective. A problem serves as a stimulus to resolve the unfulfilled value and objective. Information gathering and interpretation are mechanisms one utilizes to determine if the objectives are being met. Knowledge, skill, past experiences, and situational characteristics influence the information one gathers and the interpretations one makes of the data. General problem areas are identified from this information gathering and interpretation. This general problem area is further refined into a specific problem. This narrowing of the problem focus requires additional information processing and interpretation. More information may be needed and other data may be disregarded. As one explores a general problem area it may be evident that more than one problem exists; if this is so, then the problems are prioritized. From the general problem areas a narrower problem is identified; the components of the objective which are not being met or are threatened are determined. Next a problem statement is made; this is in the form of a question, which serves as a stimulus for the continuation of the decision making process. The problem statement asks how one can maintain the most important value in a given situation. This problem statement will serve as the basis for the search for possible solutions.

EXAMPLE 1: John Jackson

John Jackson is the head nurse of a medical-surgical unit. He has held this position for 4 years and enjoys his job. He has five children, the eldest of whom will enter college in the fall. John has recently become concerned about ability to financially support his family. Today John is told that because of a low census his unit will be closed and he can have a job as a staff nurse on a nearby unit at a reduced salary.

John suddenly feels aware of the impact of this news on himself, his family, and his job. As he thinks about this situation, he identifies and ranks his top values as:

1. Maintaining family welfare.
2. Continuing in a clinical nursing situation.
3. Increasing financial status.

His behavioral objectives for these three values are:

1. I will continually maintain the current status of family welfare by being available to my family and providing an adequate income.
2. I will continue to work in a clinical nursing situation until I retire.
3. I will strive to increase my family's financial status by exploring means of bringing in new sources of income.

To clarify the problem, John gathered the following information: his new salary, other possible jobs, costs of his child's education, and his family's feelings about this situation. He discovered: his new salary would be $100 lower per month, no jobs at his current level are presently available in his home town, his child's education will cost $1500/year, his family wants him to keep his job, and his children will apply for scholarships if possible.

John interprets this information and finds a threat to his numbers 1 and 3 values and objectives. His value of maintaining family welfare is potentially threatened by a decrease in salary. This situation also decreases his chance of increasing his financial status at this time. Thus two problems exist. The threat to maintaining family welfare is most important to John, as this is his number 1 value. This general problem is then narrowed as John evaluates his objective to see which aspect is not fulfilled or is threatened. The first objective is not being met because his ability to provide an adequate income, as defined by John, is threatened. Thus the "what" of the objective is not fulfilled. His problem is: John may not be able to provide an adequate income for his family and thus maintain family welfare. His problem statement is: "How can I maintain adequate income and family welfare in this situation?"

EXAMPLE 2: Mary and Mark

Recall the situation first presented in Chapter 4: Mary, a junior nursing student in her second day on the psychiatric–mental health rotation, is confronted with the problem of a patient, Mark, taking marijuana, alcohol, and medication.

Mary's ranked values are:

1. Maintaining life
2. Providing for physical safety
3. Maintaining a confidence

The objective for her highest ranked value is: When giving patient care I will consistently perform nursing functions that promote the maintenance of life.

At this point Mary recognizes that a problem exists. Her number 1 value and the objective derived from it are threatened by the situation. Her knowledge, skill, and past experience have helped her identify this problem. Her knowledge of pharmacology provides information she needs. Mary has had no previous experience dealing with the interaction potentials of drugs and alcohol; Mary cannot further narrow the problem at this time. Mary next assessed the validity of Mark's statements by checking with his roommates and the chart to see if this behavior had been seen previously. The roommates agreed that Mark did drink alcohol and smoke marijuana last night. His chart gives no evidence of previous attempts to tease the staff. This additional information makes her feel that the problem is a real one. Her objective, "When giving patient care I will consistently perform nursing functions that promote the maintenance of life," is threatened. Mark's life is potentially in danger due to the ingestion of drugs and alcohol.

From this information and narrowing of the problem Mary makes the following problem statement: How do I manage a potential threat to Mark's life? This problem statement is based on the threat to her objective. Mary must now find a means of removing the threat, a way to promote maintenance of life through her nursing functions.

ACTIVITIES

ACTIVITY 1
Define the term "problem" as it is used in this decision making process.

ACTIVITY 2
Read the following situation and complete the exercises.

Helen Galvin is a clinic nurse in a pediatric outpatient clinic. She likes her work with children and their families and enjoys teaching and counseling these groups. Her present position allows her to have this type of interaction with the patients and she finds her job fulfilling. Today she received a memo from her supervisor stating that the clinic will be undergoing a major change in its patient population. Adult patients will be seen in the clinic and will comprise half the patient population. Helen is to continue as clinic nurse in her present capacity.

Immediately, Helen feels upset; as her anger subsides she clarifies and ranks three values important to her at this point:
1. Working with children.
2. Doing patient teaching
3. Maintaining her current job status

Her behavioral objectives for these values are:
1. I will work professionally in the field of pediatrics as long as this field of nursing is satisfying to me.
2. Given a situation in which patient education is needed, I will provide patient teaching to the best of my ability.
3. I will maintain my current job in the pediatric clinic as long as the job fulfills my professional goals.

Helen feels there is a threat to her numbers 1 and 3 values. Before making a problem statement, Helen must determine her state of knowledge about this situation and how each of her objectives is threatened.

a. What information is known?

b. What information is needed?

c. What sources of information might Helen utilize?

ACTIVITY 3

Read the following situation and then discuss how knowledge and skill influence the recognition of a problem.

David Martin is a 2-year-old who has been hospitalized for evaluation of his short stature. This is David's first time to be away from home overnight. Last night when his mother left the hospital, David screamed and cried, not wanting his mother to leave. When she returns today she finds David is angry at her. He plays happily with the nurse, but refuses to play with his mother. Mrs. Martin is not sure what to do; she tells the aide, "I think I'll not visit tomorrow; it makes David too upset when I leave and he seems quite happy with his nurse." The aide says, "David is upset because the hospital is new to him. He'll be fine when you leave today as now he knows us." The team leader of the unit overhears this conversation and says, "David is suffering from separation anxiety. His protests are normal; it shows he cares about you. He finds it easier to express anger toward you than to us because he really fears what we might do to him."

ACTIVITY 4

Read the following situation and then describe how past experience influences the problem identification.

Alice Fowler teaches orthopedic nursing. In the "old curriculum" this course was offered as a senior specialty; this year it is to be incorporated into the second semester level medical-surgical course. For the first day of clinical experience Ms. Fowler has planned for students to do comprehensive care of two postsurgical orthopedic patients. At 10 A.M. she finds the students still reading the charts; morning care has not been started. She rushes off to coffee to think over this situation, where she complains to her fellow faculty member about "these lazy new students" who only want to do paperwork and supervise.

ACTIVITY 5

Read the following situation and then describe how situational characteristics influence problem identification.

Nancy Cannon is a new staff nurse in a convalescent hospital. She is new to the city. In the past week she and her husband have decided to separate. These life changes have left her depressed and feeling low. Today she is caring for Mr. Jones, a newly admitted stroke patient. He has spent the morning complaining about his roommate, the food, and his condition. By noon, Nancy has had it and asks for a change of assignment for the next day, saying "I don't care for Mr. Jones—he's just too uncooperative!"

ACTIVITY 6

Read the following situation and then complete the exercises.

Mary Kay Jacobson is a nurse in the labor and delivery area of a large city hospital. She also teaches childbirth preparation classes and is very excited about the trend toward family-centered obstetrical care. The unit in which she works allows fathers in the delivery room and gives parents the opportunity to have their new baby with them immediately after birth. Today Mary Kay is caring for Mr. and Mrs. Nelson, first-time parents who attended Mary Kay's prenatal classes. Mr. Nelson has been with his wife throughout her 10 hours of labor, which is now entering its final stage. He walks out of his wife's room and tells Mary Kay, "I just can't take it any more—you take care of her!" He rushes out to the waiting room. Mary feels upset and unsure about what is going on. She sees her values as:
1. Help patients successfully through labor.
2. Encourage fathers or significant others to participate in the birth experience.

3. Promote early infant-parent contact.

Her objectives for these values are:

1. I will help all patients to whom I am assigned through their labor and delivery by supporting them in. the use of childbirth preparation techniques.

2. I will encourage fathers or significant others to be actively involved in the labor and delivery process by teaching them about the process and supporting them at the time of labor and delivery.

3. I will promote early infant-parent interaction by allowing all parents to spend time with their infants immediately after birth.

a. What information does Mary Kay have at this point?

b. What information does Mary Kay need? From what sources?

c. How do knowledge, skill, past experience, and situational characteristics influence the information search, interpretation of data, and problem identification in this situation?

d. What is the general problem area?

e. What value is threatened?

f. How is the objective unfulfilled?

g. Make a problem statement for this situation.

ACTIVITY 7: Timmy: a pediatric patient

You are caring for 6-year-old Timmy, who had surgery 5 days ago. He has had several complications and his life now seems to hang by a thin thread. You have cared for Timmy since before his surgery and know it is important to his recovery to encourage him and his will to live.

This evening Timmy says to you, "Mom says John (9-year-old idolized brother) came with her tonight. He's downstairs in the lobby. I want to see him so much. I know he's not allowed to visit but please sneak him up here for just a few minutes."

In the activities in the Chapters 4 and 5 you have already:
1. Rank-ordered your values for this situation; rewrite them here:

2. Written a behavioral objective from your number 1 value; rewrite the objective here:

Your task for this chapter is to write a specific problem statement for this situation. (Be sure to consider all of the stages necessary in developing a problem statement.)

ACTIVITY 8: Fran: critical-care dilemma

You are working in critical care. Three days ago the head nurse called a staff meeting because the narcotic count had been off twice in the past 10 days. She asked all staff to be observant in the coming days for any irregularities or unexplained situations.

Today you are covering your friend Fran's patients, Mrs. Blue and Miss Snow, while Fran is at lunch. Fran said before she left that neither of them should need anything while she is gone. You stop by Mrs. Blue's bedside to check on her. She complains of pain and asks for medication. You check her chart and see that Fran has recorded meperidine (Demerol), 50 mg. IM, less than an hour ago. Mrs. Blue says she has not received a pain shot since breakfast. Puzzled, you go on to check Miss Snow and, with an uncomfortable sense of dejá vu, you have almost the same experience with her. Miss Snow is insistent that she last had pain medication before breakfast, although Fran has recorded giving Demerol within the hour.

In the activities in the previous chapters you have already:

1. Rank-ordered your values for this situation; rewrite them here:

2. Written a behavioral objective from your number 1 value; rewrite the objective here:

Your task for this chapter is to write a problem statement for this situation.

REFERENCES

1. Frederickson, K., and Mayer, G. G.: Problem solving skills: what effect does education have? Am. J. Nurs. July, 1977, pp. 1167-69.
2. Johnson, M. M., and others: Problem-solving in nursing practice, Dubuque, Iowa, 1970, Wm. C. Brown Company, Publishers.
3. McCool, B., and Brown, M.: The management response: conceptual, technical and human skills of health administration, Philadelphia, 1977, W. B. Saunders Co.
4. Rubinstein, M. F.: Patterns of problem solving, Englewood Cliffs, N. J., 1975, Prentice-Hall, Inc.
5. Monken, S. S.: After assessment—what then? Nurs. Clin. North Am. **10:** 107-120, 1975.
6. Maier, N. R. F.: Problems solving and creativity in individuals and groups. Belmont, Ca., 1970, Brooks/Cole Publishing Co.

CHAPTER

7 OPTIONS AND ALTERNATIVES

BEHAVIORAL OBJECTIVES

After completing the activities in this chapter you will be able to:

- Discuss the role of creativity in this phase of the decision making process.
- Utilize the techniques of lateral thinking, synectics, brainstorming, and quota setting in generating alternative solutions to a problem.
- Differentiate the terms "option" and "alternative" as used in this process.
- Screen the generated options in terms of meeting the stated objective to produce a list of alternatives.

This segment of the decision making process consists of two phases: generating options and screening options to identify alternatives. The goal of generating options is the production of as many potential solutions to the problem as possible. During this phase, judgment as to the feasibility, practicability, or reliability of the solution is deferred.[1] In the second phase, the options generated are screened in terms of meeting the stated behavioral objective. The options remaining are termed "alternatives" since they are alternative ways of meeting the objective.

It is suggested that "our thinking mind is mainly twofold: (1) a judicial mind which analyzes, compares and chooses; (2) a creative mind which visualizes, foresees and generates ideas."[1] The decision making process to this point has stimulated the "judicial mind" to rank values, write a behavioral objective from the top-ranked value, recognize a problem situation, and write a precise problem statement. The option generation phase has as its major focus the products of the "creative mind."

The basic concern of option generation is the quantity of options produced as opposed to the quality of each option. The rationale inherent in this statement is, of course, that the larger the number of possible solutions, the better the chances that the potentially best solution will be present.[1] When called upon to do so, one can usually produce several possible problem solutions with little effort. These usually represent routine and established modes of problem solution and do not include new and potentially better solutions. Why be concerned with new solutions to a problem when old established solutions appear to be effective? Since no two problems are exactly alike, no two solutions should have exactly the same components. In an attempt to individualize nursing actions, one needs to consider many facets of the problem in determining potential solutions. In solution generation the view of the problem and experience in creating options are possible limitations. Some people find it easy to produce new and novel ideas. The majority, however, have had very little direction in how to develop the "creative mind" and thus find it difficult to generate ideas. There are several techniques that can help develop the "creative mind" and thus increase the scope of options generated during this portion of the process. Three of these techniques are lateral thinking, synectics, and brainstorming. A fourth technique, quota setting, encourages the use of these other techniques.

LATERAL THINKING

The term "lateral thinking" was coined by Edward de Bono to describe a method for restructuring information as a means of generating new ideas.[2] "The word lateral implies moving sideways from established ways of looking at things to find new ways. This moving sideways is a search not for the best way, but for alternative ways. Traditional logical thinking is 'vertical' in nature because it takes ready made ideas and builds on them."[3] Inherent in this approach to option generation is the principle that the restructuring of information will produce alternative approaches not previously considered.

The lateral thinking approach is applicable to the decision making process; different ways of looking at the problem situation are studied in order to generate alternative approaches to the problem. For example:

"*Problem:* The problem of children getting separated from their parents in large crowds.[2]

Options might include:
1. Attach children more firmly to their parents (by a dog's lead?)
2. Better identification of children (disk with address.)
3. Make it unnecessary for children to be taken into crowds (créches, etc.)
4. Central points for parents and children to get to if losing sight of one another.
5. Display list of lost children.[2]"

Options 1 and 3 focus on ways of preventing children from being separated from their parents. The remaining options focus on ways of dealing with the problem once the separation occurs. All of the approaches were derived by restructuring the information provided in the problem situation and considering it from other perspectives.

Consider another problem and its subsequent restructuring to stimulate option generation.

Problem: The problem of patients not receiving individualized care.

If this problem is viewed with the focus on ways of providing individualized care, the following options might arise:

1. Assign one nurse to each patient for the duration of his hospitalization.
2. Develop a care plan from the patient's health history.
3. Encourage each patient to follow his usual daily routine while in the hospital.
4. Encourage each patient to make his own food selection.

If the problem is viewed with the focus of attention on ways of dealing with the patient who has not received individualized care, the options might include the following:

1. Ask the patient to discuss his expectations regarding his care.
2. Encourage the patient to discuss those aspects of his hospitalization that could have been more individualized.

Also, consider the focus of helping the nurse provide individualized care for her patients:

1. Provide the nurse with a check list covering areas of care that could be individualized (diet, personal habits, hygiene, social patterns, etc.).
2. Develop a workshop on techniques for individualizing care with the health care team.

As is apparent from the previous illustration, by restructuring and refocusing a problem situation, various options can be generated.

SYNECTICS

Synectics, like lateral thinking, involves viewing the problem from another perspective as a means of generating other ideas. Synectics is the process by which analogies are used to explore the relatedness of seemingly unrelated ideas. An analogy consists of developing one situation and comparing it to another situation, exposing the commonalities between the two. The analogous situation is developed on its own and compared at each stage of development to the problem under question. As the analogy develops, new views of the problem unfold which serve as stimuli for option generation. The major focus of synectics is on making the familiar appear strange in order to break away from a patterned way of looking at the problem. "In the 'familiar world' objects are always right-side-up; the child who bends and peers at the world from between his legs is experimenting with the familiar made strange."[4] By looking at the "familiar world" from a different vantage point the relationship of objects has changed and thus the experience has been restructured by the child, making the familiar appear different. Gordon suggests the use of analogies to make the familiar seem strange. These analogies involve either becoming personally involved with the elements of the problem, or taking some vantage point outside the problem. An illustration of projecting oneself as personally involved in the problem might be:

1. A nursing supervisor who is having problems with a particular staff member might pretend she is the staff member in order to explore ways of dealing with the situation.
2. A staff nurse in a pediatric unit who must restrain a toddler to provide a safe intravenous infusion could project herself as the toddler as a means of exploring options which might make the situation less traumatic.

The following illustrates the use of analogies as a means of generating ways of dealing with a problem and yet assuming a position outside the problem:

> A nursing staff, concerned with disturbances in the flow of communication between one shift and another, might compare this problem to what occurs when the flow of water in major tributaries is disrupted in its natural flow: (1) collateral flow may develop, bringing water to areas usually lacking water; (2) the flow is so great that the collateral flow cannot accommodate, flooding may occur.
>
> The staff could then examine whether collateral communicating channels have developed. If so, are they effective? If not, why not? Is the flow of information unchanneled or erratically channeled?

By looking at the problem from this vantage point numerous options can be generated.

BRAINSTORMING

Brainstorming is another technique designed to stimulate the creative mind to generate ideas. The term "brainstorming" means "using the brain to storm a problem."[1] Although the technique of brainstorming was originally considered a group activity, it can be used by the individual.[1] The technique consists of using one idea to stimulate another. There are numerous sources readily available as stimuli for idea production: the Yellow Pages of a telephone book, a dictionary, or a Thesaurus, to name a few.

Suppose a problem consisted of: How to make nursing care conferences more meaningful to the staff. A word randomly selected from the dictionary "equivocate" (avoid committing oneself to what one says) might stimulate the following options:

1. Keep suggestions open.
2. Tell the staff members what they would like to hear.
3. Encourage staff members to give their opinions with the freedom to modify them once given.

Or, an option once stated can be a stimulus for further option production. For example, option 3 could be the stimulus for the following options:

4. Have staff members write their suggestions on the chalk board and erase all or parts of them as they choose.
5. Have each staff member be responsible for presenting a conference on a topic of his/her choice.

Whether the brainstorming technique for option generation is used by one or many, the following rules should be followed: (1) judgement of ideas is withheld; (2) all ideas are welcome; (3)quantity of ideas is encouraged; and (4) modifying or combining ideas is encouraged.[1] By following the rules, and thus creating an environment conducive to creative option generation, you can use the technique of brainstorming to its fullest potential.

QUOTA SETTING

This technique is designed to be used in conjunction with other idea-stimulating techniques. It consists of setting a predetermined number of options to be generated. The number set should be large enough to challenge one's idea-stimulating ability. The advantage of setting a quota is that, even if one particular option appears so good that you would like to stop with it, you would have the incentive to generate more options until your quota has been met. The use of a quota is designed to be a generative technique and is not self-limiting; thus the quota set should be considered the minimum number of options to be generated and anything over the quota is strongly encouraged. The actual number set for the quota is variable and will increase as your option-generating ability improves.

•   •   •

These techniques of lateral thinking, synectics, brainstorming, and establishing a quota provide a means of generating possible solutions to the problem. All of the techniques may appear contrived and difficult to use at first, but with conscious effort they will prove to be valuable stimuli for creative option generation. It may not be possible to use each of the techniques every time the decision making process is used. Time constraints, situational characteristics, and skill in utilizing the techniques will be significant factors in determining which techniques will be selected for use.

The option generation techniques described are designed to be used in combination with each other and with the decision maker's innate ability to consider possible solutions. For example, a quota could be set on the total number of options to be generated as well as the number generated by each technique. You could start with a total quota of six, three of which may consist of solutions that immediately come to mind. Then, as a means of generating more creative solutions, the last three options can be developed through lateral thinking, synectics, or brainstorming. Regardless of how the options are generated, it is important that each is recorded, for this list is essential to the next phase of the decision making process.

THE JUDICIAL MIND

Once a list of options has been generated, the decision making process continues by calling once again on the "judicial mind" to screen for alternatives. The options are examined individually in terms of meeting the stated behavioral objective. All the options not capable of meeting the objective are rejected; the remaining options are now called alternatives. To clarify this phase consider the options that were generated earlier in this chapter regarding the problem of patients not receiving individualized care:

1. Assign one nurse to the patient for the duration of his hospitalization.
2. Develop a care plan from the patient's health history.
3. Encourage each patient to follow his usual daily routine while in the hospital.
4. Encourage each patient to make his own food selections.
5. Ask the patient to discuss his expectations regarding his care.
6. Ask the patient to discuss those aspects of his hospitalization that could have been more individualized.
7. Provide the nurse with a checklist covering areas of care that could be individualized (diet, personal habits, hygiene, social patterns, etc.).
8. Develop a workshop on techniques for individualizing care with the health care team.

If the behavioral objective is "The nurse will provide individualized care for each patient to whom she is responsible during this eight-hour shift," then options 1, 7, and 8, although possible solutions to the problem, are not capable of meeting the specific behavioral objective. These options are not possible "during this eight-hour shift" and are therefore eliminated. Those remaining options are alternative ways of meeting the behavioral objective. Further analysis of these alternatives will be the focus of the next phase of the decision making process.

SUMMARY

This chapter has discussed the creative-thinking techniques of lateral thinking, synectics, and brainstorming and the technique of quota setting as a means of generating options, possible solutions to the problem. Once the options are generated they are examined in terms of meeting the stated behavioral objective. The options not capable of meeting the stated objective are eliminated and those remaining are termed alternatives, since they are alternative ways of meeting the stated objective. This is the first judicial view of the alternatives; further analysis will continue in the next phase of the process.

EXAMPLE 1: Patrick O'Brien

Patrick O'Brien is a 63-year-old postsurgical patient who was admitted to the hospital for a bilateral radical neck surgical procedure for cancer of the larynx. He was prepared preoperatively for the fact that he would have a permanent tracheostomy and would eventually be trained in laryngeal speech. He decided he would communicate at first by writing on a Magic Slate, an eraseable pad.

Mr. O'Brien is a very independent man who prides himself on this characteristic. He owns and runs his own neighborhood bar, which he fully enjoys. He loves being with people and helping others. His four children now live in various parts of the country. His wife has had multiple sclerosis for the past 10 years and is confined to a wheelchair.

During the surgery Mr. O'Brien suffered a cerebral vascular accident; permanent blindness resulted. Now in the immediate postoperative period Mr. O'Brien cannot speak or see. His dominant arm has an intravenous infusion in it. He is currently anxious and frustrated that he cannot communicate; the independence he treasures is in great jeopardy.

Problem statement: How can I help this patient establish a communication system which would help him regain independence?

Options (quota of 7):

1. Teach the patient laryngeal speech.
2. Teach the patient Braille.
3. Set up a system of communication involving sign language.
4. Have the patient communicate by using paper and pencil, or Magic Slate.
5. Teach the patient an alphabet of textures; each texture corresponding to a different letter in the alphabet.
6. Have the patient return to his old hospital room where objects and their location are familiar.
7. Help the patient develop his nonverbal communication skills through the use of body language.

Discussion: The first four options came immediately to mind as a result of my own experience in considering similar problems. By using the lateral thinking technique of restructuring information, option 5 was created: the focus of the problem was on which of his senses were remaining as means of communication rather than which he had lost; therefore his ability to hear and touch were utilized with the textured alphabet. Option 6 reflects viewing the problem by projecting oneself as being the patient without sight or voice and wanting to be independent; by returning to a familiar environment many routine tasks could be accomplished with minimal assistance. Option 3 served as the stimulus for the creation of option 7, thus reflecting the technique of brainstorming.

Consider that the behavioral objective is: "The nurse will establish a means of communicating with Mr. O'Brien during the immediate postoperative period." This is based on the value: supporting patient independence. The initial screening of the options in terms of meeting the objective is as follows:

1. Teach the patient laryngeal speech. *Rationale:* although this may be a very good solution to the problem it will not fulfill the objective because the nurse probably does not have the skill to perform this task. Also, the time necessary to learn this technique would prohibit it from being useful in the immediate postoperative period.
2. Teach the patient Braille. *Rationale:* This option is not capable of fulfilling the objective because of skill and time restrictions.

3. Set up a system of communication involving sign-language. *Rationale:* Although formal sign language probably could not be taught by the nurse, a system involving certain hand gestures in response to questions could be developed in this time period.
4. Have the patient communiate by using paper and pencil, or Magic Slate. *Rationale:* Assuming the patient is able to write in a language that the nurse can read, this option is capable of fulfilling the stated objective.
5. Teach the patient an alphabet of textures, each texture corresponding to a different letter in the alphabet. *Rationale:* Although this option may require some time to gather various textures and place them in chart form, it can be done by the nurse in the time period and is a means of communicating.
6. Have the patient return to his old hospital room where objects and their location are familiar. *Rationale:* Although this option might promote independence for the patient, it will not fulfill the objective because it does not reflect a means of communicating.
7. Help the patient develop his nonverbal communication skills through the use of body language. *Rationale:* By using his body as a language medium, many of his needs could be communicated. This option is capable of meeting the objective because the nurse has the skill to teach Mr. O'Brien and because this can be done in the time period.

It is apparent that the *alternatives* for this situation are options 3, 4, 5 and 7.

EXAMPLE 2: Mary and Mark

Recall the situation first presented in chapter 4: Mary, a junior nursing student in her second day of psychiatric–mental health rotation, is confronted with the problem of a patient, Mark, taking marijuana, alcohol, and medication.

Mary's ranked values are:
1. Maintaining life
2. Providing for physical safety
3. Maintaining a confidence

The objective for her highest ranked value is: When giving a patient care I will consistently perform nursing functions that promote the maintenance of life.

The problem statement is: How do I manage a potential threat to Mark's life?

By using the techniques of lateral thinking, synectics, and brainstorming, the following options are evident:
1. Contact the clinical pharmacist to determine if the dosage of phenothiazines and the amount of alcohol and marijuana are harmful.
2. Say nothing and assume that the drug interaction is not harmful.
3. Give Mark Ipecac to induce vomiting.
4. Wait for signs of physical distress.

5. Call the Cardiac Arrest Team.
6. Educate Mark about the dangers of combining marijuana, alcohol, and medication.
7. Teach the nurse to be more observant when giving medication.
8. Ask the instructor for advice.
9. Tell the staff nurse about a hypothetical situation involving a patient taking marijuana, alcohol, and medication.
10. Tell the staff nurse about this situation.
11. Tell Mark about the possible interaction of drugs and find out what he would want to do.

Screening of the options in terms of meeting the behavioral objective *eliminates* the following:

Option 2: Say nothing and assume that the interaction is not harmful. *Rationale:* This does not fulfill the objective because it may not promote the maintenance of life.

Option 4: Wait for signs of physical distress. *Rationale:* Waiting for signs of physical distress may also jeopardize Mark's life.

Option 7: Teach the nurse to be more observant when giving medication. *Rationale:* Although a possible solution to the problem, this does not fulfill Mary's objective of ". . . consistently performing nursing functions that promote the maintenance of life."

Option 11: Tell Mark about the possible interaction of drugs and find out what he would want to do. *Rationale:* This would not fulfill Mary's objective if Mark chose not to maintain his life.

Therefore, the following alternatives exist for Mary: options 1, 3, 5, 6, 8, 9, and 10.

ACTIVITIES

These activities are designed to help you review the content of the chapter and to meet the objectives.

ACTIVITY 1
Discuss the role of the "creative mind" and the "judicial mind" in this phase of the decision making process.

ACTIVITY 2
Define the following techniques and give an example of each.

Lateral thinking:

Synectics:

Brainstorming:

Quota setting:

ACTIVITY 3
Define and differentiate the terms "option" and "alternative" as used in this process.

ACTIVITY 4
The following activity will give you practice in screening options to identify alternatives.

Behavioral objective: I will continually maintain the current status of family welfare by being available to my family and providing an adequate income.

Problem statement: How can family welfare be maintained?

Options:
1. Get a new job with higher salary.
2. Maintain several jobs to ensure adequate income.
3. Reduce expenses to ensure adequacy of income.
4. Encourage others in the family to provide financial assistance.

Circle the workable alternatives and state why each of the remaining options is not an alternative.

•   •   •

The following activities are designed to provide practice in using all of the components of the decision making process learned to this point.

ACTIVITY 5: Henry: a patient with COPD
It is the seventh hospital day for Henry Stills, a 68-year-old male with a history of chronic obstructive pulmonary disease (COPD) and cor pulmonale. He is a 100-pack/year smoker and has not had a cigarette since the day of

admission. This is the third admission to the unit this year for Henry because of acute respiratory distress as a result of recurrent pulmonary infections.

Henry's condition has greatly improved since admission. He has resumed all of his daily activities, his current respiratory infection appears to be resolving, and he will probably be discharged within a day or two. You are the staff nurse who has been taking care of Henry during this admission and through several of the previous admissions. As you come in Henry's room to make morning rounds you find Henry sitting in bed smoking a cigarette; and you also notice six cigarette butts discarded in a paper cup at the bedside.

a. What values would you have in this situation? Rank them.

b. Write a behavioral objective from your top-ranked value.

c. After examing the problem situation:
   (1) Identify information that is known.

   (2) Identify information that is unknown and may be valuable.

   (3) Write a problem statement.

d. Generate six options, three of which reflect the techniques of lateral thinking, synectics, and brainstorming.
   (1)
   (2)
   (3)
   (4)
   (5)
   (6)

e. After screening the options in terms of meeting your stated behavior objective, list the possible alternatives for this situation.

ACTIVITY 6: Timmy: a pediatric patient

You are caring for 6-year-old Timmy, who had surgery 5 days ago. He has had several complications and his life now seems to hang by a thin thread. You have cared for Timmy since before his surgery and know it is important to his recovery to encourage him and his will to live.

This evening Timmy says to you, "Mom says John (9-year-old idolized brother) came with her tonight. He's downstairs in the lobby. I want to see him so much. I know he's not allowed to visit but please sneak him up here for just a few minutes."

In the activities in the previous chapters you have already:
1. Rank-ordered your values for this situation. Rewrite them here:

2. Written a behavioral objective from your number 1 value. Rewrite the objective here:

3. Written a problem statement for this situation. Rewrite it here:

Your task for this chapter is to:
a. Generate options for this situation. Write them here:

b. Screen the options to determine possible alternatives. List them here:

ACTIVITY 7: Fran: critical-care dilemma

You are working in critical care. Three days ago the head nurse called a staff meeting because the narcotic count had been off twice in the past 10 days. She asked all staff to be observant in the coming days for any irregularities or unexplained situations.

Today you are covering your friend Fran's patients, Mrs. Blue and Miss Snow, while Fran is at lunch. Fran said before she left that neither of them should need anything while she is gone. You stop by Mrs. Blue's bedside to check on her. She complains of pain and asks for medication. You check her chart and see Fran has recorded meperidine (Demerol), 50 mg. IM, less than an hour ago. Mrs. Blue says she has not received a pain shot since breakfast. Puzzled, you go on to check Miss Snow and, with an uncomfortable sense of deja vu, you have almost the same experience with her. Miss Snow is insistent that she last had pain medication before breakfast, although Fran has recorded giving Demerol within the hour.

In the activities in the previous chapters you have already:

1. Rank-ordered your values for this situation. Rewrite them here:

2. Written a behavioral objective from your number 1 value. Rewrite the objective here:

3. Written a problem statement for this situation. Rewrite it here:

Your task for this chapter is to:

a. Generate options for this situation. Write them here:

b. Screen the options to determine possible alternatives. List them here:

REFERENCES

1. Osborn, A. F.: *Applied imagination,* New York, 1963, Charles Scribner's Sons, pp. 39, 124, 142, 151, 156.
2. de Bono, E.: *Lateral thinking: creativity step by step,* New York, 1970, Harper and Row, Publishers, p. 14, 87, 88.
3. de Bono, E.: *PO: A device for successful thinking,* New York, 1972, Simon and Schuster, p. 94.
4. Gordon, W. J. J.: *Synectics: the development of creative capacity,* New York, 1961, Harper & Row, Publishers, p. 35.

8 ANALYZING ALTERNATIVES

After completing the activities in this chapter you will be able to:

- Identify the three criteria used in analyzing alternatives.
- Define in your own words the concepts of desirability, probability, and personal risk taking.
- Analyze and rank each of the alternatives in terms of desirability, probability, and personal risk, given an actual or hypothetical situation.

As you enter this stage of the decision making process, you are equipped with a set of possible alternatives. Each alternative has the potential of solving the problem under consideration; that is, all alternatives are capable of meeting the objective, alleviating the threat to the value system and thus restoring equilibrium.

How then do you select from these alternatives? Many selection methods are possible. You could use a trial and error approach, starting with the first alternative and proceeding to try each alternative individually; this may result in eventual success but is time consuming and may cause you frustration. Another approach might be to rely on your intuition. Many great scientists have done just this, but the majority of nursing decisions cannot wait for intuition.

The best approach requires an analysis of all alternatives. Each can be judged by specific criteria. This results in a systematic approach applicable for all individual decisions.

Three major criteria are utilized for analyzing alternative solutions; these are desirability, probability, and personal risk taking. Each of these criteria may assume a different degree of importance for a particular problem. In one situation, desirability may be the main criterion; in another, probability or risk taking may be most important. The use of these criteria enables you to examine each alternative in a systematic manner. All three must be utilized for effective alternative analysis.

DESIRABILITY

The first criterion is desirability, which can be defined as a subjective measurement of the individual's preference for an alternative. Desirability is influenced by several major factors: the particular situation at hand, values, situational constraints such as time or resources, institutional policies and procedures, patient characteristics, and the nurse's knowledge, skill, and past experience. What is the most desirable alternative for you may not be the most desirable for another individual. Desirability will also change for you at various times. If you are hungry you may find food very desirable; when your appetite is satiated, food may lose its desirability. Desirability, then, is situation-dependent—it allows you a choice as to what is most important to you at *that* moment for *that* problem. Desirability is determined by your value system. Thus, as you screen alternatives you can identify those that best express your values at that point.

The concept of desirability has its origins in utility theory. ". . . utility is defined as want-satisfying power. According to the principles of utility theory, the rational decision maker calculates deliberately and chooses consistently, always with a view toward maximizing his utility. The maximization of utility means that the decision maker makes those choices that will result in his having the greatest possible amount of satisfaction."[1] This theory is used in economic and business management decision theory. For these disciplines utility is a measure of satisfaction which is expected to come from an alternative. This satisfaction frequently reflects that of a collective or corporation, often in dollar value. Complex mathematical formulas are applied, or payoff tables are utilized to select the best alternative. This measure of utility requires that one is able to quantify decision outcomes. While this may be possible in some situations, most nursing decisions cannot be reduced to a mathematical formula. The facts that nursing is an applied science and that many nursing decisions involve applying information or skills which must be adjusted for the specific patient reduce the applicability of a quantitative approach. It is true that research may define appropriate intervention techniques but the decision to utilize them with a particular patient in a certain circumstance requires a nursing decision.

Desirability may also be influenced by features other than values. Although all alternatives are possible solutions, you must consider the desirability for this specific situation. Such considerations include constraints of the situation as well as positive and negative aspects of the alternative. Constraints might include resources such as equipment or workload. For example, an alternative which involves the use of equipment not currently present on the unit may be less desirable than an alternative which uses resources presently available to the nurse. Also, an alternative which would consume more time than is currently available to the nurse, thus requiring reassignment or overtime, might be less desirable than an alternative which can be carried out in a shorter time. The ability of the nurse may serve as a positive or negative influence. If the nurse is unsure of a certain procedure, its desirability may decrease; if, however, the nurse is confident in this skill, desirability may increase.

A hospital policy or procedure may influence the desirability of an alternative. The nurse's policy manual might state guidelines for patient care within an institution, or a job description might specifically state activities you must do to fulfill your position. Both of these policies would influence your determination of desirability. If the nurse is rewarded for patient teaching, the desirability of such an alternative may increase. Policies may dictate the desirability of alternatives by clarifying those areas of care that will result in reward for the nurse.

Time may influence desirability, as may the short-term or long-term considerations. Do you have sufficient time to carry out a particular alternative, or are you in a rush to care for other patients or finish other duties? Also, it is possible that the short-term or immediate aspects of an alternative may be desirable but future effects are not very preferable. An alternative may commit you, the decision maker, to future activities which you may not desire. For example, choosing not to study for a test may be desirable to an overloaded student, but she may end up having to put in extra effort at a later time in order to master the content.

If the nursing decision directly involves a patient, then the characteristics and preferences of that patient must be considered as an influence on desirability. An alternative may decrease or increase in desirability if considered in terms of a particular patient.

> For example, consider the dilemma of Margaret Blumberg, a staff nurse in a convalescent hospital. She is caring for John Thomas, a 32-year-old paraplegic with severe decubitus ulcers. Margaret realizes that Mr. Thomas' nutritional state is very important to his recovery. A high-protein diet has been ordered. Margaret also knows that Mr. Thomas is a dedicated vegetarian. Margaret is to help Mr. Thomas plan his meals. She sees his menu has the following food selections: roast beef sandwich, lasagna, peanut butter sandwich, hamburger, and a vegetable plate. To help Mr. Thomas have an adequate nutritional input, Margaret sees three alternatives: (1) select the food for Mr. Thomas, (2) let him order the food and hope he selects the appropriate ones, and (3) select the food with Mr. Thomas. The alternatives have different desirability for Margaret as she takes into consideration Mr. Thomas' particular characteristics, as well as the time she has to spend with him. By selecting the food for Mr. Thomas she could pick the highest protein food, yet she would be ignoring his personal preferences. Letting him select his food is Margaret's normal preference, but in this case Mr. Thomas' nutritional state must receive higher consideration than usual. Selecting the food with Mr. Thomas is the most desirable, as she can meet his personal preferences

and at the same time ensure a high-protein diet; in other words, he could order a peanut butter sandwich with milk and receive complete protein. Thus alternatives may increase or decrease in desirability, depending on the particular patient.

A system for ranking desirability must be developed for each problem situation. Each alternative needs to be ranked for desirability, and no two alternatives should have the same ranking. For example, in a situation with three alternatives three degrees of desirability are needed: highly desirable, moderately desirable, and least desirable. This ranking will be individually determined by you. The alternative which is most desirable is the highest ranked, alternatives of medium desirability are placed in the middle, and those least desirable are at the end. Ranking forces you to make a determination of all the alternatives as to desirability and will become important in your final alternative selection. In some situations all alternatives may seem of equal desirability or none may seem desirable. Ranking will require you to sort these out, to look carefully at the factors influencing the situation. This analysis will help you determine a desirability ranking for alternatives in any situation.

The following example demonstrates the use of desirability in analyzing alternatives.

> Alice Jones, a staff nurse, is responsible for caring for Mrs. Brown, a postoperative patient. It is near the time for shift change when Mrs. Brown complains of pain in her surgical site. Alice clarifies three of the possible alternatives: (1) medication, (2) communicating with Mrs. Brown about her pain, and (3) positioning Mrs. Brown.

Alice clarifies three values that are inherent in her objective: "To provide optimal patient care within the eight-hour shift for my assigned patients." These values are (1) getting off work on time, (2) patient comfort, and (3) responsibility to others. She sets these values in the following priority:
1. Responsibility to others
2. Getting off work on time
3. Patient comfort

In ranking these alternatives according to desirability, Alice would make the following determination:

Possible alternatives	Desirability ranking
Medication	Highly desirable 1
Communicating with Mrs. Brown	Least desirable 3
Positioning Mrs. Brown	Moderately desirable 2

Her rationale might sound like this: Medicating Mrs. Brown allows me to finish my duties and give report to the oncoming shift. They are not delayed in their work and I have taken care of meeting my responsibility to others. Talking to

Mrs. Brown is the least desirable, as it involves time, which would make me late giving report and would interfere with the work of the next shift. This choice would also make me late getting off work, even though it might make Mrs. Brown more comfortable. Positioning Mrs. Brown would be rated as moderately desirable, for it would take less time than talking to Mrs. Brown and more time than medicating her. By positioning her I would delay the report and also might get off work late.

Now consider Maria Hernandez, a staff nurse with the same behavioral objective in this situation. Her values are ranked: (1) patient comfort, (2) responsibility to others, and (3) getting off work on time. Utilizing the same alternatives she would rank her alternatives for desirability as: talking to Mrs. Brown, highly desirable; positioning Mrs. Brown, moderately desirable; and medicating Mrs. Brown, least desirable.

How would you rank the three alternatives as to desirability if your values were ranked: (1) getting off work on time, (2) patient comfort, and (3) responsibility to others?

PROBABILITY

The alternatives under consideration are further analyzed in terms of probability, that is, the likelihood of an event occuring. The event under consideration in the decision making process is the success of the alternative; probability can be defined in this context as the likelihood that the alternative will be successful and meet the objective.

Much of probability theory has dealt with objective probabilities, the frequent example being the toss of the coin. Given that one side of a coin is a head and the other side is a tail and the coin is tossed, there is a 50 percent chance that the coin will land with the tail showing and likewise there is a 50 percent chance that the coin will land with the head showing. Accordingly, the probability of the coin coming up heads is 50 percent. Objective probabilities are of particular value in routine and recurrent choices whose frequencies have been observed in numerous trials. Unfortunately, this has very little application in the analysis of alternatives that have to do with human choice and thus is of little significance to the individual decision maker.

On the other hand, subjective probability is a very valuable criterion in the analysis of human decision. Subjective probability is the rating that the individual places on the likelihood that the alternative will be successful. As with the selection of alternatives, an individual's subjective probability of any one choice is based on his past experience, present information, and situational constraints. The numerical value you place as your probability rating is individually determined. An alternative that you feel will be highly successful would be rated 75 percent or above. Those with a 50 percent chance of success and a 50 percent chance of failure would be given a 50 percent rating. Alternatives which you feel have a low chance of success would be rated below 25 percent. The particular situation and your values, past experience, knowledge, and skill will enable you to rank the alternatives in terms of probability. Since very few decisions deal with either complete certainty (100 percent probability) or complete uncertainty (0 percent probability), most decisions will be rated between 1 and 99. In the decision process presented in this book only subjective probabilities are considered. Therefore the alternative of "medicating" was given the highest probability of success, "communicating" the lowest probability of success, and "positioning" an equal probability of success and failure. What probability rating would you assign to each of the alternatives given the same information?

Alternatives (in rank order)	Probability
1. Medicate	80%
2. Communicate	10%
3. Position	50%

1. When the patient had been given medication previously, the pain subsided quickly.
2. Positioning in the past had been successful in about as many times as it has been unsuccessful.
3. The patient is predominantly Spanish speaking and, even though Alice speaks a little Spanish, her vocabulary is not extensive enough to converse with the patient in the time permitted.

Therefore the alternative of "medicating" was given the highest probability of success, "communicating" the lowest probability of success, and "positioning" an equal probability of success and failure. What probability rating would you assign to each of the alternatives given the same information?

PERSONAL RISK TAKING

Personal risk taking is the third criterion utilized for analyzing possible alternatives. "Risk" can be defined as "hazard" or "exposure to chance of injury, damage or loss."[2] Risk involves an evaluation of the hazards of a selected solution in relation to the benefits of that solution.[3] The criterion of personal risk taking represents an individual's analysis of the alternatives in terms of hazard versus benefit for a particular problem situation. As with the other two criteria, desirability and probability, the rating of risk by the decision makers is based on his past experiences, present information, and situational constraints. An alternative may be highly desirable and have a high probability of success and at the same time pose too much risk for the decision maker.

The concept of personal risk has three dimensions: (1) physical risk (2) emotional risk, and (3) social risk.[3] Although these three elements are usually combined in an individual's evaluation of risk, it is helpful for you to be aware of the composition of each of the elements. Physical risk may be viewed as a potential or actual threat to body integrity which may occur to you and/or your patient. For example, you might hurt your back attempting to lift an obese, comatose patient, or you might be pregnant and not wish to risk caring for a baby with congenital rubella. You consider the physical risk to patients in many circumstances: ambulation, feeding, and giving medications are but a few. You might pose physical risk to a suicidal patient by leaving him alone. Aspiration might result from early initiation of tube feeding in a patient with weak swallow and gag reflexes. Physical risk is a daily part of nursing and must be carefully analyzed in each situation.

Emotional risk may result from a threat to one's psychological being or self-concept. This risk may also involve you and/or your patient. It may be a risk for both you and your patient to discuss his need for becoming more independent. You may like serving his needs and he may feel it is not fair to make him do tasks which are painful, or which he can no longer do as well as he once did. Working with people results in many emotional risks. You are exposed psychologically; this may cause you to face feelings and beliefs you do not wish to face. The same is true for your patient. Illness may result in changes in his self-concept. Seeking health care might make him feel he is dependent on others, or he might discover he needs to change certain aspects of his way of life. All these situations involve emotional risk, a common occurrence in health care delivery situations.

Social risk refers to a threat to one's role in society, that is, one's position and function. Social risk is also frequently found in your interactions with patients. You may find your role as a nurse, woman, male, student, parent, or other challenged by your job or patient. As a student, you might face the patient who does not want "any student nurses caring for me!" As a graduate, you might face a patient who prefers the other nurse because "she knows just how to do it right." Such situations put your roles in society at risk. Patients also face social risk. The 40-year-old executive who has his first myocardial infarction faces risks to his role as parent, spouse, provider, and male, to name a few. The mother whose child is failing to thrive is presented with risks to her roles as woman and mother. Social risks are often found in nursing situations and must be considered in the total evaluation of risk.

These three elements of risk can be considered individually or in combination. All elements may or may not be present in a given situation. Your goal is to make a determination of the risk of a situation. Whether you do this by considering each dimension of risk separately or by viewing risk as a combination of elements is not important. The objective is to determine ranking of risk for the alternative under scrutiny.

Alternatives can be ranked as high, moderate, or low risk. The rating is subjective as the determination is done by the individual and is situation-dependent.

Up to now the concept "risk" has been presented. Personal risk taking as a criterion for analyzing alternatives encompasses more than risk determination.

Even though risk-taking behavior may be a personality component, the situation will influence how much risk the individual is willing to assume at that time. For example, a nurse who works in a critical care unit may not view taking a central venous pressure reading as a risky procedure. A beginning student may rank this same procedure as high-risk. Thus, knowledge and skill may determine risk. This relationship may go in either direction. The more knowledge you have about an alternative, the more risks you may identify; or, knowledge may decrease risk interpretation. Risk is situation-dependent for many nursing decisions.

Your values may also influence personal risk taking. To meet a value of high priority, you may be willing to assume more risk. A working knowledge of your values allows you to determine the amount of risk you are willing to take to fulfill this value. A problem situation which involves a value of very high priority for an individual may call for more risk taking. Consider the situation in which cardiopulmonary resuscitation (CPR) is an alternative. It is highly probable that the CPR maneuver will produce some physical injury to the patient, whether this be a fractured rib or bruised sternum. If you value maintaining life above possibly inflicting injury on another, you would decide to do CPR despite the risk involved.

The following situation demonstrates the rating of personal risk taking. In reference to the patient situation involving Alice Jones and Mrs. Brown, Alice's values are ranked: (1) responsibility to others, (2) getting off work on time, and (3) patient comfort. In her analysis of the three alternatives Alice finds the following risks:

Alternatives	Risk evaluation
1. Medicating Mrs. Brown	High physical risk
2. Communicating with Mrs. Brown	Moderate emotional and social risk
3. Position Mrs. Brown	Moderate physical risk

If Alice sees physical risk as a greater risk than emotional or social risk, she would rank the alternatives accordingly:

Alternatives	Risk ranking
Medication	High 1
Communicating	Low 3
Positioning	Moderate 2

It can be seen that although the three dimensions of risk might be analyzed initially, an overall risk ranking is the final result, representing the overall risk of that particular alternative. No two alternatives can have the same risk ranking.

In the above situation, assume that Alice sees emotional/social risk as high risk, what might her risk ranking be for these alternatives?

SUMMARY

This chapter has dealt with three criteria used in analyzing alternative solutions: desirability, probability, and personal risk. Desirability, which has its origins in utility theory, is the criterion that measures the individual's preference for an alternative. Subjective probability is the rating that the individual places on the likelihood that the alternative will be successful. Risk represents an individual's analysis of the alternatives in terms of hazards versus benefits of a particular problem situation. Each of the criteria is rated for each alternative in question.

All three of these major criteria must be used to analyze any alternative. There may be times when none of the alternatives seems desirable, yet it is essential that ranking be done. The same is true for risk taking. All alternatives may appear to have the same risk, yet differentiation between the alternatives for levels of risk is vital. Probabilities should also differ for each alternative. As stated earlier, any one criterion may assume top priority in consideration for a given situation, yet all three criteria must be utilized for alternative analysis. Systematic decision making requires analysis of all alternatives by desirability, probability, and risk taking. The next step in the decision making process will be based on this complete alternative analysis.

EXAMPLE: Mary and Mark

Recall the situation (first presented in Chapter 4) of Mary, a junior nursing student in her second day of the psychiatric–mental health rotation, confronted with the problem of a patient, Mark, taking marijuana, alcohol, and medication. Mary's ranked values are:

1. Maintaining life
2. Providing for physical safety
3. Maintaining a confidence

The objective for her highest ranked value is: When giving patient care I will consistently perform nursing functions that promote the maintenance of life.

The problem statement is: How do I manage a potential threat to Mark's life?

Options were generated and screened in chapter 7 to identify alternatives. An analysis of the alternatives consists of the following:

Alternative 1: Contact the clinical pharmacist to determine if the dosage of phenothiazine and amounts of alcohol and marijuana are harmful.
Desirability: very high.
Rationale: it may determine that no problem exists.
Probability: high, 75 percent.
Rationale: with accurate information the exact threat would be known, and the exact medical regime could be recommended.
Personal risk: moderate overall.
Rationale: low physical (very little physical risk to either Mark or Mary); high emotional risk (due to threat of breaking a confidence with Mark); moderate social risk (some embarrassment involved in asking pharmacist).

Alternative 3: Give Mark Ipecac to induce vomiting.
Desirability: moderate.
Rationale: it is an intrusive procedure which may prove unnecessary.
Probability: low, 25 percent.

Rationale: time has passed since the ingestion of alcohol and drugs, reducing the effectiveness of this approach.

Personal risk: high overall.

Rationale: moderate physical risk (Mark may aspirate vomitus); high emotional and social risks for Mary (her role as a student, as well as the nurse-patient relationship is threatened).

Alternative 5: Call the cardiac arrest team.

Desirability: low.

Rationale: a cardiac arrest may not occur.

Probability: low, 10 percent.

Rationale: Unless Mark has a cardiac arrest the team will not be helpful.

Personal risk: very high overall.

Rationale: low physical risk to Mary and Mark but high for other patients (the team is not available for them if needed); high emotional and social risks to Mary and Mark (as a result of calling attention to the situation).

Alternative 6: Educate Mark about the dangers of combining marijuana, alcohol, and medication.

Desirability: high.

Rationale: when considering long-term effect, this alternative is desirable.

Probability: very low, 5 percent.

Rationale: will not help Mark at this time (threat already exists).

Personal risk: very low overall.

Rationale: low physical risk (cannot harm Mary or Mark); low emotional and social risks (Mark gave the information and Mary is sharing her knowledge with him).

Alternative 8: Ask the instructor for advice.

Desirability: high.

Rationale: instructor can maintain confidence with student.

Probability: moderate, 50 percent.

Rationale: it will take time to discuss the situation, decreasing its chance for success.

Personal risk: moderate overall.

Rationale: low physical risk (little physical harm will come to Mark or Mary as a result of this); moderate emotional and social risk (Mary may fear that the instructor may expect a higher level of knowledge from her).

Alternative 9: Tell the staff nurse about a hypothetical situation involving a patient taking marijuana, alcohol, and medication.

Desirability: low.

Rationale: would rather be open and honest about the situation.

Probability: low, 15 percent.

Rationale: several factors contribute to this: time, accuracy of information, and validity of the staff nurse's response (since she believes it to be a hypothetical situation).

Personal risk: overall low.

Rationale: less risk involved than in the real situation.

Alternative 10: Tell the staff nurse about this situation.
   Desirability: moderate.
      Rationale: more desirable than Alternative 9 (can be open and honest).
   Probability: low, 20 percent.
      Rationale: slightly higher than Alternative 9 because staff nurse may have more knowledge and past experience that could apply.
   Personal risk: low-moderate overall.
      Rationale: this involves more emotional and social risk than telling instructor because another person is involved who may not maintain a confidence with Mark.

The previous analysis is summarized in Table 1.

TABLE 1. Analysis of alternatives

Alternative	Desirability (highest, 1; lowest, 7)	Probability (percent)	Risk (highest, 1; lowest, 7)
1. Contact clinical pharmacist to determine if the dosage of phenothiazine and the amount of alcohol and marijuana are harmful	Very high 1	High 75	Moderate 4
3. Give Mark Ipecac to induce vomiting	Moderate 4	Low 25	High 2
5. Call cardiac arrest team	Low 7	Low 10	Very high 1
6. Educate Mark about the dangers of combining marijuana, alcohol, and medication	High 3	Very low 5	Very low 7
8. Ask instructor for advice	High 2	Moderate 50	Moderate 3
9. Tell the staff nurse about a hypothetical situation involving a patient taking marijuana, alcohol, and medication	Low 6	Low 15	Low 6
10. Tell the staff nurse about this situation	Moderate 5	Low 20	Low-moderate 5

ACTIVITIES

These activities are designed to review the content of this chapter.

ACTIVITY 1

Define: "desirability," "probability," and "personal risk taking."

ACTIVITY 2: John James: hospitalized 2-year old

You are a nurse on a pediatric unit. It is time for you to give John James his early-evening antibiotic injection. John has been hospitalized for three days. His mother is able to visit only in the evenings. This has created separation anxiety in John and he becomes frantic when his mother leaves. John also becomes upset when he gets his injection. His mother is not sure how to help John when he gets his shot and is willing to go along with your suggestions. You have no choice about whether or not to give the medicine. You have proceeded with the decision making process. The following alternatives have resulted from screening options:

1. Ask Mrs. James to wait outside the room and come in immediately after the medication is given.
2. Allow Mrs. James to stay in the room and help restrain John.
3. Allow Mrs. James to stay in the room and have another nurse help restrain John.
4. Send Mrs. James to have her dinner.

Complete the following activities. The accompanying form may be helpful to you.

a. Rank the desirability of the alternatives.

b. State those factors which influenced your desirability ranking.

c. State the probabilities for the alternatives. (What factors influenced your rating?)

d. Rank the risk in the above situation. State the factors which influenced your ranking.

e. How would your ranking change if alternatives 2 and 3 are against accepted policy on the pediatric unit?

Alternative	Desirability (most desirable, 1; least desirable, 4)	Probability (percent)	Risk (highest, 1; lowest, 4)
Ask Mrs. James to wait outside the room and come in immediately after the medication.			
Allow Mrs. James to stay in the room and help restrain John.			
Allow Mrs. James to stay in room and have another nurse help restrain John.			
Send Mrs. James for her dinner.			

ACTIVITY 3: Timmy: a pediatric patient

You are caring for 6-year-old Timmy who had surgery 5 days ago. He has had several complications and his life now seems to hang by a thin thread. You have cared for Timmy since before his surgery and know it is important to his recovery to encourage him and his will to live.

This evening Timmy says to you, "Mom says John (9-year-old idolized brother) came with her tonight. He's downstairs in the lobby. I want to see him so much. I know he's not allowed to visit but please sneak him up here for just a few minutes."

In the activities in the previous chapters you have already:

1. Rank-ordered your values for this situation. Rewrite them here:

2. Written a behavioral objective from your number 1 value. Rewrite the objective here:

3. Written a problem statement for this situation. Rewrite it here:

4. Made a list of possible alternatives. List them here:

Your task for this chapter is to rank each alternative in terms of desirability, probability, and personal risk. Consider the factors which influenced your ranking.

ACTIVITY4: Fran: critical-care dilemma

You are working in critical care. Three days ago the head nurse called a staff meeting because the narcotic count had been off twice in the past 10 days. She asked all staff to be observant in the coming days for any irregularities or unexplained situations. Today you are covering your friend Fran's patients, Mrs. Blue and Miss Snow, while Fran is at lunch. Fran said before she left that neither of them should need anything while she is gone. You stop by Mrs. Blue's bedside to check on her. She complains of pain and asks for medication. You check her chart and see that Fran has recorded meperidine (Demerol), 50 mg. IM, less than an hour ago. Mrs. Blue says she has not received a pain shot since breakfast. Puzzled, you go on to check Miss Snow and, with an uncomfortable sense of deja vu, you have almost the same experience with her. Miss Snow is insistent that she last had pain medication before breakfast, although Fran has recorded giving Demerol within the hour.

In the activities in the previous chapters you have already:
1. Rank-ordered your values for this situation. Rewrite them here:

2. Written a behavioral objective from your number 1 value. Rewrite the objective here:

3. Written a problem statement for this situation. Rewrite it here:

4. Made a list of possible alternatives. List them here:

Your task for this chapter is to rank each alternative in terms of desirability, probability, and personal risk. Consider the factors which influenced your ranking.

REFERENCES

1. Harrison, F. E.: *The managerial decision making process*, Boston, 1975, Houghton-Mifflin Co. p. 226.
2. Guralnik, D. B. editor: *Webster's New World Dictionary,* Second College Edition, Cleveland, 1974 William Collins and World Publishing Co., Inc.
3. Clarke, K., and Parcel, G. S.: Values and risk-taking behavior: the concept of calculated risk, Health Education, November-December, 1975, pp. 26-28.

9 MAKING THE DECISION

After completing the activities in this chapter you will be able to:

- Examine the problem situation under consideration and determine which of the analysis criteria (desirability, probability, personal risk) are of particular significance.
- Compare each alternative in terms of the priorities identified in the problem situation (i.e., behavioral objective 1).
- Choose the alternative that best correlates with priorities established from the problem situation.
- Evaluate the chosen alternative in terms of the decision making process.

The next step in the decision making process is the selection of the alternative solution to be utilized. The systematic decision making process makes this step a relatively easy one. A clear value, a behavioral objective, and a set of alternatives that are well analyzed are prerequisite to this step. From the alternatives you must now choose one that will best meet the behavioral objective, thus fulfilling the value in question for the problem situation. By now you must certainly be asking how this final selection is done. Fortunately or unfortunately, depending on your values, there is no set rule that is applicable for all decisions. There is, however, a means of further analyzing the problem situation that will help you in the selection of the best alternative for a particular situation.

ANALYSIS OF THE PROBLEM SITUATION

The original problem situation is now analyzed to see which of the three criteria utilized for alternative analysis is most important; that is, the criteria—

desirability, probability, and personal risk taking—are placed in priority for the problem at hand. This ranking of the three criteria is situation-dependent and changes continually for the individual decision maker over time. For a certain situation the desirability of the alternatives may be so important that probability and risk taking seem less important or even unimportant. In another situation an alternative having a high probability for success may be the most important. Any combination of these three criteria can be utilized as the basis for selecting the best alternative.

The analysis considers all three criteria, which are then ranked. This analysis may show you that one criterion has an overwhelming priority. The alternative that best meets this criterion is then selected. For example, if upon reexamination of the problem situation you see desirability is most important to you, then the alternative with the highest desirability should be selected. If, on the other hand, you believe that the situation requires a low-risk, high-probability alternative and that desirability is insignificant, then an alternative that best fits that description is picked.

To clarify this phase, reconsider the situation involving Alice Jones, a staff nurse, responsible for caring for Mrs. Brown, a postoperative patient (Chapter 8).

PROBLEM SITUATION

Time of shift change when Mrs. Brown complains of pain in surgical site.

ALTERNATIVE ANALYSIS

	Desirability	Probability	Risk
1. Medicate	High 1	High 80%	High 1
2. Communicate	Moderate 2	Low 10%	Low 3
3. Position	Low 3	Moderate 50%	Moderate 2

Suppose you return to the problem situation and determine by your analysis that desirability and probability are of major significance and risk is of little significance. Thus it is important for you to make a decision that is highly desirable personally and with a high probability of success, regardless of the risk; therefore, you would choose the alternative "medicate." If, however, upon analysis of the problem situation you determine that risk is of major significance, you would choose the alternative "communicate." This would be the alternative with the least amount of risk involved, with moderate desirability, and with a very low probability of being successful. You would choose the alternative "position" if you thought that the probability and risk criteria were of equal importance and desirability was of little significance.

Thus the priorities established from the original problem situation dictate which of the possible alternatives would be most reflective of your personal values inherent in the problem situation, as well as the behavioral objectives derived from those values.

FACTORS INFLUENCING ALTERNATIVE SELECTION

Alternative selection is a personal matter. Which criterion is seen as most important will vary from person to person. What makes the three criteria assume different priorities for different situations? This is a complex question, for priority ranking is based on many factors. The value that is threatened certainly influences the ranking of criteria. A value that is of high priority may result in a totally different ranking of the criteria than a value of lower priority. Remember the example of cardiopulmonary resusitation? The value operating at that time, maintaining life, may be of high priority to the nurse. Thus, she might rank alternatives using probability as the criterion of top priority (probability of success being more important than risk taking or desirability).

Knowledge of the situation and past experiences also influence the ranking. For example, a nurse who has had experience working with a particular patient might arrange the ranking of the criteria in a different order than the nurse who has had no such experience. The past experience or knowledge of the situation might make desirability and probability more important than risk taking. Or, on the other hand, risk taking may be more carefully determined based on past experiences with certain interventions. For instance, the nurse who has performed cardiopulmonary resuscitation (CPR) several times on the same patient over the past eight hours may consider risk the most important criterion influencing her choice not to perform CPR again on that patient.

Present situational factors such as time, resources, and policies are also important considerations. For example, a nurse who is operating with limited resources may rank probability higher than risk or desirability. She may need to select an alternative with a high probability of success because of her lack of resources. She may be willing to take a high risk and is less concerned about desirability in this situation.

Personality characteristics may also influence the ranking. Some individuals tend to consistently avoid risk; thus they might always seek to select alternatives of low risk.

A GOOD DECISION

You may ask, "How do I know that the alternative I choose represents a good decision?" A good decision is derived from all phases of the decision making process, which has values clarification as its base. It may be viewed as the apex of a pyramid, with the composite layers being the other phases of the process, each one building on the other. If the alternative selected is derived from all of the building elements, then it is a good decision. (See the figure on p. 103.)

EVALUATION

Evaluation of the decision is the next stage in this process. As has been stated previously, a good decision is not the same as a good outcome. The decision is

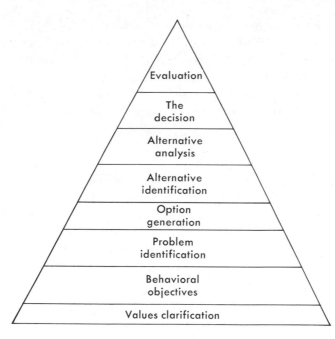

judged by whether or not the systematic process was utilized, not by the outcome alone.

One method of determining whether the decision reflects all of the previous stages of the process is to reexamine the previous phases in light of the decision, by asking yourself the following questions:

1. Does the decision, analyzed in terms of desirability, probability, and personal risk, correlate with the priority areas assessed in the problem?

   If it does not—return to the list of analyzed alternatives and select one that coincides.

   If it does—continue with the evaluation by considering the next question.

2. Does the decision reflect your stated behavioral objective?

   If it does not—return to the alternative analysis phase and consider the remaining alternatives.

   If it does—continue with the evaluation by considering the final question.

3. Does your behavioral objective reflect your priority value for this situation?

   If it does not—restate the behavioral objective to reflect the value.

   If it does—the decision is derived from all of the building elements and is by definition a good decision.

You may ask, "What if I evaluate the decision all the way back to the value clarification phase and decide that I no longer agree with my value ranking?" Then you must start the process again, this time with the new priority value. But keep in mind that the process, as described, is situation-dependent; a time lapse may mean that upon reexamination you find that your value ranking and priorities have changed. This change may be the result of a different value that is threatened; thus a new problem exists and the decision process begins again.

As has been stated earlier, a good decision is the result of systematic use of this process. Once you are able to apply this process to a problem, good decisions will result. Good decisions imply that you have made systematic choices based on your value system.

SUMMARY

This chapter focuses on making the decision. The analyzed alternatives are compared with the significant components of the problem situation. The alternative that best reflects the priorities suggested by the problem situation is the alternative of choice.

Evaluation, the final phase of the process, involves a reexamination of all the previous phases.

EXAMPLE: Mary and Mark

Recall the situation (first presented in Chapter 4) of Mary, a junior nursing student in her second day of the psychiatric—mental health rotation, confronted with the problem of a patient, Mark, taking marijuana, alcohol, and medication. Mary's ranked values are:

1. Maintaining life
2. Providing for physical safety
3. Maintaining a confidence

The objective for her highest ranked value is: When giving patient care I will consistently perform nursing functions that promote the maintenance of life.

The problem statement is: How do I manage a potential threat to Mark's life?

Options have been generated and screened to identify alternatives. These alternatives have been analyzed as summarized in Table 2.

Upon reexamination of the problem situation, it is determined that "probability" is the most important criteria. In this instance, Mary wants an alternative that has the highest probability of success. She is least concerned with the "desirability" of the alternative and moderately concerned with the "risk" involved.

Mary's decision is to contact the clinical pharmacist to determine if the dosage of phenothiazine and the amount of alcohol and marijuana is harmful—alternative 1. This alternative best correlates with Mary's ranking of the criteria for the problem situation. When evaluating the decision Mary considers the following questions:

1. Does the decision, analyzed in terms of desirability, probability, and personal risk, correlate with the priority areas assessed in the problem? Yes.
2. Does the decision reflect your stated behavioral objective? Yes.
3. Does your behavioral objective reflect your priority value for this situation? Yes.

Mary's decision is derived from all elements of the process and is by definition a good decision! (See Table 3 for a summary of the decision making process in the example of Mary and Mark.)

TABLE 2. Analysis of alternatives

Alternative	Desirability (highest, 1; lowest, 7)	Probability (percent)	Risk (highest, 1; lowest, 7)
1. Contact clinical pharmacist to determine if the dosage of pheno-thiazine and the amount of alcohol and marijuana are harmful.	Very high 1	High 75	Moderate 4
3. Give Mark Ipecac to induce vomit-ing.	Moderate 4	Low 25	High 2
5. Call cardiac arrest team.	Low 7	Low 10	Very high 1
6. Educate Mark about the dangers of com-bining marijuana alcohol, and medi-cation.	High 3	Very low 5	Very low 7
8. Ask instructor for advice.	High 2	Moderate 50	Moderate 3
9. Tell the staff nurse about a hypothetical situation in-volving a patient taking marijuana, alcohol, and medication.	Low 6	Low 15	Low 6
10. Tell the staff nurse about this situation.	Moderate 5	Low 20	Low-moderate 5

ACTIVITIES

ACTIVITY 1: a family in stress

Abe Jones is a 2-year-old white male who was admitted to the Pediatric ICU 3 days ago with pneumonia. The medical work-up confirmed the diagnosis of, "cystic fibrosis (C.F.) with secondary pneumococcal pneumonia." Abe is the youngest of three children. One brother, John, is 4 years old and is in good health. A 6-year-old brother, Billy, died last summer in the same Pediatric ICU following an unsuccessful rescue attempt by the paramedics after the youngster was found in the bottom of a swimming pool.

The Jones' have been divorced for a year. Mr. Jones keeps no contact with his family. All extended family members live at least 500 miles away. Mrs. Jones has taken on the full support of the family by working as a waitress.

TABLE 3. Summary of decision making process in the example of Mary and Mark

1. Values in rank order	2. Behavioral objective	3. Problem statement	4. Options
1. Maintaining life 2. Providing for physical safety 3. Maintaining a confidence	When giving patient care I will consistently perform nursing functions that promote the maintenance of life.	How do I manage a potential threat to Mark's life.	1. Contact the clinical pharmacist to determine if the dosage of phenothiazines and the amount of alcohol is harmful. 2. Say nothing and assume that the drug interaction is not harmful. 3. Give Mark Ipecac to induce vomiting. 4. Wait for signs of physical distress. 5. Call the cardiac arrest team. 6. Educate Mark about the dangers of combining marijuana, alcohol, and medication. 7. Teach the nurse to be more observant when giving medications. 8. Ask the instructor for advice. 9. Tell the staff nurse about a hypothetical situation involving a patient taking marijuana, alcohol, and medication. 10. Tell the staff nurse about this situation. 11. Tell Mark about the possible interaction of drugs and find out what he would want to do.

5A. List of alternatives	5B. Analysis of alternatives (highest, 1; lowest, 7)			6. Problem situation (highest, 1; lowest, 3)			7. Decision	8. Evaluation	If yes, go to next question	If no, return to step
	Desirability	Probability (percent)	Personal risk	Desirability	Probability	Personal risk				
1. Contact the clinical pharmacist to determine if the dosage of phenothiazine and the amount of alcohol and marijuana are harmful	1	75	4	3	1	2	Alternative 1: Contact the clinical pharmacist to determine if the dosage of phenothiazine and the amount of alcohol and marijuana are harmful	1. Does the decision, analyzed in terms of desirability, probability and personal risk, correlate with the priority areas assessed in the problem?	yes	5B
3. Give Mark Ipecac to induce vomiting	4	20	2							
5. Call the cardiac arrest team	7	10	1							
6. Educate Mark about the dangers of combining marijuana, alcohol and medication	3	5	7					2. Does the decision reflect your stated behavior objective?	yes	5A
8. Ask the instructor for advice	2	50	3					3. Does your behavioral objective reflect your priority value for this situation?	yes	2
9. Tell the staff nurse about a hypothetical situation involving a patient taking marijuana, alcohol, and medication	6	15	6							
10. Tell the staff nurse about this situation	5	20	5							

The nurses in the Pediatric ICU are becoming concerned about Mrs. Jones' interaction with Abe; they have noticed the following behaviors: (1) she visits twice a day although visiting hours are unrestricted, (2) she stays with Abe for only 5 to 10 minutes a visit, (3) while with Abe, she insists the nurse be present with her, (4) she focuses her attention on the equipment, not on Abe; she does not speak with Abe or provide physical contact, and (5) she frequently calls Abe by his dead brother's name.

The Pediatric ICU utilizes primary care nursing. One nurse is assigned to the patient upon admission and follows him until discharge. She is to perform an initial assessment and develop a plan of care, which is utilized by all nurses caring for the patient. The care plan is comprehensive as the unit philosophy emphasizes parental education and discharge planning. This planning begins on admission, and parents are encouraged to participate and learn about their child's care throughout his ICU stay.

Because of Abe's diagnosis, cystic fibrosis, it is important to teach Mrs. Jones postural drainage and percussion at this time. You are Abe's primary care nurse and you must decide how to incorporate Mrs. Jones into Abe's care. Your values are:

Parent participation and education
Individualized care
Nonstressful patient care unit
Family as patient unit
Responsibility to parents' needs

These values are ranked:

1. Individualized care
2. Parent participation and education
3. Family as the patient unit
4. Responsibility to parents' needs
5. Nonstressful patient care unit

The *behavioral objective* for the priority value is: You (the nurse) will provide individualized care for Abe at all times while caring for him in the pediatric ICU by considering Abe and his mother and brother's present and long-term needs.

The *problem statement* is: How to prepare the mother with the knowledge and skill required for Abe's discharge?

The following *options* for the problem are generated:

1. Refer Mrs. Jones for psychotherapy.
2. Ask Mrs. Jones if she wishes to participate in Abe's care.
3. Ask Abe how he wants his mother included in his care.
4. Intervene with Mrs. Jones' anxiety prior to any parent teaching efforts.
5. Bring in an extended family member to take care of Mrs. Jones' emotional needs.
6. Continue to teach Mrs. Jones despite her anxiety.
7. Have another C. F. parent, rather than the nurse, teach Mrs. Jones in the Pediatric ICU.

8. Set up a plan of care which gradually involves Mrs. Jones in Abe's care.
9. Send Mrs. Jones to a C. F. parent group for education before returning to the Pediatric ICU to care for Abe.
10. Put Mrs. Jones on diazepam (Valium) and then take her into the room for teaching.
11. Call the supervisor and ask her to intervene with Mrs. Jones.
12. Ask the staff nurse who worked with Mrs. Jones at the time of Abe's brother's death what techniques were successful in working with Mrs. Jones.
13. Ask that Abe be transferred to another hospital where parents do not participate in their child's care.

Those options that do not fulfill the behavioral objective are eliminated:
1. Refer Mrs. Jones for psychotherapy.
2. Ask Abe how he wants his mother included in his care.
5. Bring in an extended family member to take care of Mrs. Jones' emotional needs.
7. Have another C. F. parent, rather than the nurse, teach Mrs. Jones in the Pediatric ICU.
9. Send Mrs. Jones to a C.F. parent group for education before returning to the Pediatric ICU to care for Abe.
10. Put Mrs. Jones on Valium and then take her into room for teaching.
11. Call the supervisor and ask her to intervene with Mrs. Jones.
13. Ask that Abe be transferred to another hospital where parents do not participate in the child's care.

This leaves you with the following alternatives, which are then ranked or rated for desirability, probability and risk taking in Table 4.

a. As Abe's primary care nurse, rank the criteria of desirability, probability, and risk taking for this problem situation.

b. Select the alternative which best fits your criteria ranking for this problem situation.

c. Use the evaluation process to evaluate your decision.
   (1) Does the decision, analyzed in terms of desirability, probability, and personal risk, correlate with the priority areas assessed in the problem? If it does not, return to the list of analyzed alternatives and select one that coincides.

TABLE 4. Ranking of alternatives

Alternative	Desirability (highest, 1; lowest, 5)	Probability (percent)	Risk (highest, 1; lowest, 5)
1. Ask Mrs. Jones if she wishes to participate in Abe's care.	4	50	1
2. Intervene with Mrs. Jones' anxiety prior to any parent teaching efforts.	1	80	3
3. Continue to teach Mrs. Jones despite her anxiety.	5	5	2
4. Set up a plan of care which gradually involves Mrs. Jones in Abe's care.	2	60	4
5. Ask the staff nurse who worked with Mrs. Jones at the time of Abe's brother's death what techniques were successful in working with Mrs. Jones.	3	35	5

If it does, continue with the evaluation by considering the next question.

(2) Does the decision reflect the stated behavioral objective?

If it does not, return to the alternative analysis phase and consider the remaining alternatives.

If it does, continue with the evaluation by considering the final question.

(3) Does the behavioral objective reflect the priority value for this situation?

If it does not, restate the behavioral objective to reflect the value.

If it does, the decision is derived from all the building elements and is by definition a good decision.

ACTIVITY 2: Timmy: a pediatric patient

You are caring for 6-year-old Timmy who had surgery 5 days ago. He has had several complications and his life now seems to hang by a thin thread. You have cared for Timmy since before his surgery and know it is important to his recovery to encourage him and his will to live. This evening Timmy says to you, "Mom says John (9-year-old idolized brother) came with her tonight. He's downstairs in the lobby. I want to see him so much. I know he's not allowed to visit but please sneak him up here for just a few minutes."

In the activities in the previous chapters you have already:

1. Rank-ordered your values for this situation. Rewrite them here:

2. Written a behavioral objective from your number 1 value. Rewrite the objective here:

3. Written a problem statement for this situation. Rewrite it here:

4. Made a list of possible alternatives. List them here:

5. Ranked each alternative in terms of desirability, probability, and personal risk. Write your rankings here:

Your task for this chapter is to:

a. Rank desirability, probability, and personal risk for the problem situation:

b. State your decision:

c. Evaluate your decision:

(1) Does the decision, analyzed in terms of desirability, probability, and personal risk, correlate with the priority areas assessed in the problem?
    If it does not, return to the list of analyzed alternatives and select one that coincides.
    If it does, continue with the evaluation by considering the next question.
(2) Does the decision reflect your stated behavioral objective?
    If it does not, return to the alternative analysis phase and consider the remaining alternatives.
    If it does, continue with the evaluation by considering the final question.
(3) Does your behavioral objective reflect your priority value for this situation?
    If it does not, restate the behavioral objective to reflect the value.
    If it does, the decision is derived from all of the building elements and is by definition a good decision.

ACTIVITY 3: Fran: critical-care dilemma

You are working in critical care. Three days ago the head nurse called a staff meeting because the narcotic count had been off twice in the past 10 days. She asked all staff to be observant in the coming days for any irregularities or unexplained situations. Today you are covering your friend Fran's patients, Mrs. Blue and Miss Snow, while Fran is at lunch. Fran said before she left that neither of them should need anything while she is gone. You stop by Mrs. Blue's bedside to check on her. She complains of pain and asks for medication. You check her chart and see that Fran has recorded Demerol, 50 mg. IM, less than an hour ago. Puzzled, you go on to check Miss Snow and, with an uncomfortable sense of deja vu, you have almost the same experience with her. Miss Snow is insistent that she last had pain medication before breakfast, although Fran has recorded giving Demerol within the hour.

In the activities in the previous chapters you have already:

1. Rank-ordered your values for this situation. Rewrite them here:

2. Written a behavioral objective from your number 1 value. Rewrite the objective here:

3. Written a problem statement for this situation. Rewrite it here:

4. Made a list of possible alternatives. List them here:

5. Ranked each alternative in terms of desirability, probability, and personal risk. Write your rankings here:

Your task for this chapter is to:
a. Rank the problem situation in terms of desirability, probability, and personal risk:

b. State your decision:

c. Evaluates your decision:
   (1) Does the decision, analyzed in terms of desirability, probability, and

personal risk, correlate with the priority areas assessed in the problem?

If it does not, return to the list of analyzed alternatives and select one that coincides.

If it does, continue with the evaluation by considering the next question.

(2) Does the decision reflect your stated behavioral objective?

If it does not, return to the alternative analysis phase and consider the remaining alternatives.

If it does, continue with the evaluation by considering the final question.

(3) Does your behavioral objective reflect your priority value for this situation?

If it does not, restate the behavioral objective to reflect the value.

If it does, the decision is derived from all of the building elements and is by definition a good decision.

CHAPTER
10 PUTTING IT ALL TOGETHER

BEHAVIORAL OBJECTIVE

After completing the activities in this chapter you will be able to:

■ Apply the decision making process presented in this book to actual or hypothetical situations, utilizing all of the components.

The purpose of this section to is to provide you with clinical situations in which to practice the decision making process. Following each situation is a format to guide you with the process.

SITUATION 1

You are a school nurse in an urban high school. The mother of the star of the basketball team, Jeff Zabruiski, has just called you to request a home teacher for Jeff for the rest of the school year. Jeff had a grand mal seizure two weeks ago, his first such seizure, He had been hospitalized for a complete work-up. He was diagnosed as having "Seizure disorder—etiology unknown." He is now home and is on seizure medications. He has had no further seizures. Mrs. Zabruiski tells

1. Values (in rank order)	2. Behavioral objective	3. Problem statement	4. Options	5. Alternatives			
				A. List	B. Analyzed		
					Desirability	Probability	Personal risk

you she wants Jeff to stay home until he's "well." She says she and his father have convinced Jeff not to go away to college next year and that he must give up his hopes for a basketball scholarship. She says being around his friends will only depress Jeff and that a home teacher is the only answer. When you requested to speak to Jeff you were told "he's resting." According to school policy Jeff is eligible for a home teacher, but the final determination is up to you.

What decision would you make?

6. Problem situation			7. Decision	8. Evaluation	If *yes,* go to next question	If *no,* return to step
Desirability	Probability	Personal risk				
				1. Does the decision, analyzed in terms of desirability, probability, and personal risk, correlate with the priority areas assessed in the problem?		5B
				2. Does the decision reflect your stated behavior objective?		5A
				3. Does your behavior objective reflect your priority value for this situation?		2

SITUATION 2

You are a public health nurse making a routine newborn visit at the Williams' home. Mrs. Williams had been discharged from the local medical center 1 week ago after delivering her fourth child, David, a full-term, eight-pound, healthy boy. As you are examining David you observe that Mrs. Williams seems quite tired and withdrawn and that the house is in a state of upheaval. The three other children stay away from you, frequently running into see their father who is in the front bedroom watching television, drinking beer, and demanding numerous errands

1. Values (in rank order)	2. Behavioral objective	3. Problem statement	4. Options	5. Alternatives A. List	B. Analyzed Desirability	Probability	Personal risk

by the children. As you approach the other children you see they all have numerous bruises. One child appears to have a burn on his hand. As you question Mrs. Williams about your observations, she does not seem to have answers and seems more apprehensive. At that time Mr. Williams comes out and wants to know why you are asking all the questions. . . . "You came to see David; you did, and that's that! You've completed the newborn examination." What decision would you make?

6. Problem situation					If *yes*, go to next question	If *no*, return to step
Desirability	Probability	Personal risk	7. Decision	8. Evaluation		
				1. Does the decision, analyzed in terms of desirability, probability, and personal risk, correlate with the priority areas assessed in the problem?		5B
				2. Does the decision reflect your stated behavior objective?		5A
				3. Does your behavior objective reflect your priority value for this situation?		2

SITUATION 3

You are the evening supervisor of three busy medical units in a large hospital; you have held this position for 3 years. The job is very satisfying and has resulted in good rapport with the nursing staff. Prior to becoming a supervisor, you worked as a staff nurse on one of these units for 5 years. Six months ago primary care nursing became the method for giving patient care in the hospital. In the past, team nursing and functional assignments had been utilized. An extensive in-service program was carried out to teach the staff the method of primary care. At first the method was enthusiastically utilized by the personnel. You observed the results of better patient teaching and fewer patient and physician complaints. You strongly feel this is an excellent method of giving patient care. Lately you have noticed many of the evening nurses have returned to functional nursing.

1. Values (in rank order)	2. Behavioral objective	3. Problem statement	4. Options	5. Alternatives A. List	B. Analyzed Desirability	Probability	Personal risk

They tell you that functional nursing is much less trouble for them as it is less time-consuming. Your efforts to convince them to continue with primary care have not been successful. The staff is becoming increasingly upset with you. They say they have tried but the new method just will not work. The director of nursing wants a full-year trial of this program and is relying on you to make this a successful project. This concerns you, as supervisors are directly responsible to the director of nursing in this hospital. You are hoping to become an associate director soon but are also becoming more frustrated as a result of the declining staff rapport and your obviously diminishing authority. The staff wants you to make an exception in their case: let them go back to their previous ways of giving care. What decision would you make?

6. Problem situation				8. Evaluation	If *yes*, go to next question	If *no*, return to step
Desirability	Probability	Personal risk	7. Decision			
				1. Does the decision, analyzed in terms of desirability, probability, and personal risk, correlate with the priority areas assessed in the problem?		5B
				2. Does the decision reflect your stated behavior objective?		5A
				3. Does your behavior objective reflect your priority value for this situation?		2

SITUATION 4

Kim is a mental health nurse employed by the county. As a member of the crisis team she evaluates individuals for voluntary and involuntary hospitalization. By state law, individuals are hospitalized involuntarily for psychiatric evaluation when they are an immediate danger to themselves or others or when, for mental reasons, they are unable to provide for their own food, shelter, and clothing.

The sheriff's department has asked the crisis team to evaluate Mrs. Stuart. She calls the sheriff frequently for imagined thefts and she has been seen by the sheriff eating from garbage cans. When Kim arrives she finds Mrs. Stuart out walking. Mrs. Stuart greets Kim pleasantly and asks her in. The house is dusty and in disarray; not one chair is empty to sit in. The smell is musty. Kim asks to look around the house. Mrs. Stuart walks with her from room to room. She is talking about her husband not being home. This makes her sad and she hopes he

1. Values (in rank order)	2. Behavioral objective	3. Problem statement	4. Options	5. Alternatives			
				A. List	B. Analyzed		
					Desirability	Probability	Personal risk

will soon be home; she is waiting. Kim knows from the sheriff that Mr. Stuart died a year ago. The bathroom is flooded with water. Mrs. Stuart says the toilet broke last week. The refrigerator has several colonies of mold and one onion inside. The sink is filled with crusted dishes. Kim asks Mrs. Stuart when she last ate. "This morning, I made some beans," was her reply.

As Kim continues to look around and talk with Mrs. Stuart, Kim mentally reviews the literature she has been reading on separation and aging. Research underlines the severity of the effects of sudden, involuntary separation from home on the health and life expectancy of older people. Kim thinks of the large, understaffed state hospital where Mrs. Stuart would be sent if she is involuntarily hospitalized.

Putting yourself in Kim's place, complete your evaluation of Mrs. Stuart. What decision would you make?

Desirability	Probability	Personal risk	7. Decision	8. Evaluation	If *yes*, go to next question	If *no*, return to step
6. Problem situation						
				1. Does the decision, analyzed in terms of desirability, probability, and personal risk, correlate with the priority areas assessed in the problem?		5B
				2. Does the decision reflect your stated behavior objective?		5A
				3. Does your behavior objective reflect your priority value for this situation?		2

SITUATION 5

Linda teaches psychiatric–mental health nursing on a progressive inpatient psychiatric unit. The nurses there assume responsibility for group therapy and other extended role functions. Linda personally values the roles these nurses fulfill and often talks with students about the professional values involved. Linda holds responsibility and accountability as both personal and professional values.

In the course of post–group discussion one afternoon Linda listened as one of her students described a troubling group experience. The description ended with the statement that one of the nurse-therapists, Arlene, had fallen asleep twice

As the instructor, what decision would you make?

1. Values (in rank order)	2. Behavioral objective	3. Problem statement	4. Options	A. List	Desirability	Probability	Personal risk

Table header spanning: **5. Alternatives** over (A. List and B. Analyzed); **B. Analyzed** spanning Desirability, Probability, Personal risk.

during the group therapy session. Linda's expression registered disbelief and anger before she validated that the happenings in the group were indeed disturbing.

As a nursing instructor who must continue teaching in this unit, Linda considers that she needs to respond to Arlene's sleeping in the group. If you put yourself in Linda's position, what decision would you make? If you were the student and your instructor said it was your responsibility to deal with the situation, what decision would you make?

6. Problem situation			7. Decision	8. Evaluation	If *yes*, go to next question	If *no*, return to step
Desirability	Probability	Personal risk				
				1. Does the decision, analyzed in terms of desirability, probability, and personal risk, correlate with the priority areas assessed in the problem?		5B
				2. Does the decision reflect your stated behavior objective?		5A
				3. Does your behavior objective reflect your priority value for this situation?		2

Situation 5 format continued on pp. 126-127.

As the student, what decision would you make?

1. Values (in rank order)	2. Behavioral objective	3. Problem statement	4. Options	5. Alternatives A. List	B. Analyzed Desirability	Probability	Personal risk

6. Problem situation			7. Decision	8. Evaluation	If *yes*, go to next question	If *no*, return to step
Desirability	Probability	Personal risk				
				1. Does the decision, analyzed in terms of desirability, probability, and personal risk, correlate with the priority areas assessed in the problem?		5B
				2. Does the decision reflect your stated behavior objective?		5A
				3. Does your behavior objective reflect your priority value for this situation?		2

SITUATION 6

You are an industrial nurse in a large electronics plant. You have been employed there for the past 2 years and routinely work during the day. For this week only you are working evenings.

Shortly after your shift begins, 46-year-old Mr. Azula comes into the clinic office assisted by a co-worker. Mr. Azula is holding a clenched fist over his sternum and complaining of tight, squeezing pain radiating into his left shoulder and down his left arm. Mr. Azula is perspiring and pale. He complains of difficulty breathing and nausea. As you take his wrist to feel his pulse, you observe that his hands are cool and moist. His pulse is 96, his blood pressure is 100/70.

1. Values (in rank order)	2. Behavioral objective	3. Problem statement	4. Options	5. Alternatives			
				A. List	B. Analyzed		
					Desirability	Probability	Personal risk

You pull his folder and note that twice in the past 3 weeks Mr. Azula has been taken from work to the community hospital emergency room with suspected myocardial infarction. On both occasions he was released with a diagnosis of acute anxiety attack. Mr. Azula's pulse was recorded as 86 and 88 and his blood pressure was 122/80 and 115/80 on these two visits. After the second visit to the emergency room, Mr. Azula was referred to a mental health clinic. What decision would you make?

6. Problem situation						
Desirability	Probability	Personal risk	7. Decision	8. Evaluation	If *yes*, go to next question	If *no*, return to step
				1. Does the decision, analyzed in terms of desirability, probability, and personal risk, correlate with the priority areas assessed in the problem?		5B
				2. Does the decision reflect your stated behavior objective?		5A
				3. Does your behavior objective reflect your priority value for this situation?		2

SITUATION 7

You are a staff nurse in a ten-bed intensive care unit. One of your patients is Herbert Williams, a 45-year-old male who was admitted several days ago for active gastrointestinal bleeding. Upon admission to the unit there was a moderate amount of bright red blood from his nasogastric tube that subsided within 20 minutes with continuous iced saline lavage. Since there has not been a recur-

1. Values (in rank order)	2. Behavioral objective	3. Problem statement	4. Options	5. Alternatives			
				A. List	B. Analyzed		
					Desirability	Probability	Personal risk

rence of the bleeding episode, Mr. Herbert's nasogastric tube was removed. A medical order has been written to transfer him to the fourth floor, where he will undergo an extensive medical workup. As you are preparing Mr. Williams for transfer he directs your attention to an emesis basin containing 50 ml of a bright red substance which he stated he vomited 10 minutes earlier. What decision would you make?

Desirability	Probability	Personal risk	7. Decision	8. Evaluation	If *yes*, go to next question	If *no*, return to step
6. Problem situation						
				1. Does the decision, analyzed in terms of desirability, probability, and personal risk, correlate with the priority areas assessed in the problem?		5B
				2. Does the decision reflect your stated behavior objective?		5A
				3. Does your behavior objective reflect your priority value for this situation?		2

EPILOGUE

PATIENT INVOLVEMENT

The focus of this book has been on the nurse as the decision maker. Most nursing decisions, however, involve patients. Patients are a very important part of this decision making process. Nurses no longer "do for" or "do to" patients. Patients' involvement in their own care is an essential component of successful nursing care. This need for patient involvement in the decision making process is emphasized by nursing education and becomes a highly held professional value. Patient involvement, that is, the patient's view and his way of life, is incorporated into the nurse's values. Values such as "patient comfort" or "patient safety" are individualized in this process. For example, "patient comfort" for your patient Mrs. Anderson must take into consideration her personality characteristics and life situation: a 90-year-old widow who dislikes medications and prefers backrubs and conversation.

Values which affect patient care are learned. Sociology, psychology, and anthropology can help the nurse expand her understanding of people. These theories, in addition to medical and nursing knowledge, are applied to individual patients so that priorities in care can be established for the individual patient. The patient must never be lost sight of in the decision making process if effective care is to be given.

There may be occasions when your personal values are ranked higher than those values which are patient-oriented, or when your values and patient values conflict. The process of value conflict resolution will hopefully reduce any disturbance you might encounter as a result. If this is not possible, it is vital that you find another resource that can meet the patient's need. For example, suppose "parental care for children" is a strong value that you hold—you are outraged by child abuse. You are assigned to care for Steve Bilkes, a 4-year-old who was physically abused by his mother. You discover you cannot stand being in the room when she arrives. You are angry and want to hit her. Yet you know she is in need of help and that parent involvement is a high value of your patient unit. It is necessary that you find another resource for Mrs. Bilkes. Nurses are people. Times will occur when your values must come first, but the patient must not suffer as a result. By recognizing such unresolved conflicts you can plan alternatives which will benefit you and the patient.

The process presented in this book demonstrates the importance of values. Patients are a major part of the nurse's value system and thus are included throughout the process. The definition of the problem situation will reflect these values which are unmet. The criteria utilized for analyzing the alternatives and the problem situation are highly influenced by values. You, as a nurse, hold values which are patient-based; therefore, the patient becomes an integral part of this decision making process.

TEACHING THE DECISION MAKING PROCESS

This decision making process is a helpful tool that can be taught to patients, co-workers, and peers. Teaching this process is not complex since people learn by observation and experience. You can serve as a role model for your patients and co-workers and are in an ideal situation to teach this process. They can see you put the process into action, and thus observe the decision making process. You can work with individual patients on a problem they face. Begin by helping the patient identify pertinent values. He then can rank the values and develop a behavioral objective. The problem situation is then stated. The patient can form options and determine which options are realistic alternatives for him. He can be helped to analyze the alternatives and the problem situation, making the final choice of alternatives himself. Evaluation of the decision can then be carried out.

Going through the process step by step will not only lead to the patient solving the problem, he will also learn a process that will equip him to make future decisions. Work groups can also learn this process; this will help the individual members as well as the group as a whole.

DECISION MAKING IN GROUPS

Thus far this book has addressed only personal, individual decision making. The authors recognize that nurses work primarily in groups, as members of a team. This is true of staff nurses in hospitals and clinics, as well as nurses in supervisory positions. Even nurses working alone in offices and schools work in collaboration with others. When nurses do make decisions alone, others are likely to be involved in implementing the decisions.

Nurses also work with patient groups. Although a particular patient may be the focus, nurses work with families. Hospital and community nursing can be family-centered. Nurses also work with non-family groups of patients. Rehabilitation and therapy groups are common in psychiatric nursing.

Working with groups inevitably means decision making with groups. Therefore, this epilogue includes a summary of group dynamics as they are related to decision making and a discussion of the advantages and disadvantages of group decision making. The decision making process described in this book is applicable to group decisions as well as individual decisions. The differences in the process are those which are brought about by the dynamics of the group.

Nurses work in two different types of groups. Ongoing groups are established groups which meet together over time; a head nurse group, a cardiopulmonary resusitation team, or the maternal-child health interest group of the state nurses' association are examples of established groups. Ad hoc groups meet together for a particular purpose, then disband; a discharge planning meeting with a family is such a group.

The dynamics of the two types of groups are different because of the differences in time. There are likely to be differences in the importance of the group to its members and in committment to the group. Regardless of differences, knowledge of group dynamics is helpful in understanding group behavior and your role in the group. When you understand group forces and your position, you are better able to make constructive contributions to the group and choose to accept alternatives without feeling you have compromised yourself or been manipulated by subtle social pressures.

A group is considered a group when it has particular characteristics. Two or more people who identify themselves and can be identified as members of the group are prerequisite. The group must have a common purpose and be able to act as a single unit. Members interact within the group and are interdependent on one another to meet their needs and goals.[1] Individual members will be committed to the group to the extent that the group meets their needs and goals and they feel accepted by the group. Individual committment to the group, along with cohesiveness and cooperation within the group, are ingredients for a successfully functioning group.

A clear, agreed-upon goal is a chief determinant of group effectiveness. Agreement on means to reach this goal and the investment of individual energies by each member into this group goal are then needed. The organization of the group, coordination of tasks, and availability of resources also influence effectiveness. The effectiveness of any group can be enhanced by the process of examining and discussing the current group process and by trying new ways.[1]

Conflict in groups refers to the different response tendencies elicited in various members from a single situation—it does *not* mean interpersonal hostility. Conflict often enhances the effectiveness of an ongoing group; conflict increases the number and discussion of alternatives considered without being perceived as a threat to the group or as hostility to members. The result of conflict is likely to be a creative, workable solution. Conflict disrupts the minimal committment and cohesion in an ad hoc group. If a unique solution is arrived at, it is likely to be a compromise less workable than already proposed alternatives.[2]

The advantages of group decisions can be summarized as the possibility of better decisions and better implementation. Several appropriate individuals necessarily have broader experience and a wider range of knowledge than a single individual. This means a greater number of options and consequences can be identified by a group and analyzed from several critical viewpoints. Research findings support the superiority of a group's final decision over the average individual's alternative solution.[2]

Disadvantages of group decision making include time and social pressures. It takes more time for a group to discuss alternatives and arrive at a consensus than for an individual to make a decison. This process may be frustrating to task-oriented members. The dynamics of the group may include social pressure toward conformity. If an individual sees his position as subordinate in a group and/or if the group has great value to him, he will be more vulnerably to group pressures toward conformity. "Groupthink" is the name given by Janis to the process of individual group member's suppressing their own critical thinking and questioning of an alternative. This happens when the individual has internalized a group norm for agreement and values agreement more highly than thorough consideration of alternatives.[3]

The diffusion of responsibility that occurs with group versus individual decisions may be an advantage or a disadvantage. Individuals within a group may be more open to a variety of possible solutions because the possibility of personal criticism is lessened.

Shifts in choice, especially risky choices, are a possible disadvantage of group decision making. The process of group decision making may support individual members taking a more extreme position and course of action than they would take individually.[4] Thus, there is the possibility of unnecessary risk or unhelpful conservatism from a group decision.

Participation in and shared responsibility for a decision has the advantage of leading to a greater understanding of and committment to the final choice. This is especially helpful when the group responsible for the decision is also responsible for implementation.

Leader and member roles may be a disadvantage in decision making. Some patterns of leadership, especially disorganized leadership which lacks direction, may contribute to difficulty in the group decision process. Group member roles which center attention on the individual, rather than the group and its task, are a hindrance to decision making. Individual group members who do not understand the decision making process can also hamper group decision making.

Some types of decisions are more advantageously made in groups, while others are more effectively made by individuals. Harrison summarizes the characteristics of decisions most effectively and efficiently made by individuals as routine, recurrent decisions which have a degree of certainty. Decisions which are neither routine nor recurrent or predictable are best made in a group. He suggests that group decision making is an advantage in setting objectives because of the broader knowledge base. Evaluating alternatives within a group is also an advantage because of the broader range of critical analysis available.[5]

To make group decisions or not make group decisions is not a relevant question. Nurses work in groups and make decisions in groups. How to maximize the group process of decision making is a relevant question. A general understanding of group dynamics and your roles in groups is the first step. Then, an awareness of the advantages of group decision making will help you to gain the most from the situation. An awareness of the disadvantages will help you to recognize and minimize these pitfalls. Finally, group discussion of your own group process will enhance the process and the decision making outcome.

REFERENCES

1. Knowles, M., Knowles, H.: Introduction to group dynamics, New York, 1972, Association Press, pp. 40-41, 63-64.
2. Hall, J.: Decisions, decisions, decisions, Psychology Today, November, 1971, pp. 51-53.
3. Janis, I. L.: Groupthink, Psychology Today, November, 1971, p. 43.
4. Main, E. C., and Walker, T. G.: Choice shifts and extreme behavior: judicial review in the federal courts, Soc. Psychol. **91**:215, 1973.
5. Harrison, F. E.: The managerial decision making process, Boston, 1975, Houghton-Mifflin Co., pp. 210-214.